How to Quickly and Accurately Master ECG Interpretation

DALE DAVIS, RCT
ECG Supervisor and Computerized ECG
  Systems Manager
Morristown Memorial Hospital
Morristown, New Jersey

Illustrated by Patrick Turner

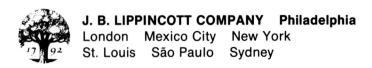

J. B. LIPPINCOTT COMPANY   **Philadelphia**
London   Mexico City   New York
St. Louis   São Paulo   Sydney

How to Quickly and Accurately Master ECG Interpretation

Acquisitions Editor: Lisa A. Biello
Sponsoring Editor: Delois Patterson
Manuscript Editor: Lauren McKinney
Indexer: Ann Cassar
Art Director: Tracy Baldwin
Design Coordinator: Anne O'Donnell
Designer: Patrick Turner
Production Supervisor: Kathleen Dunn
Production Coordinator: George V. Gordon
Compositor: Bi-Comp, Inc.
Printer/Binder: R. R. Donnelley & Sons Company
Cover Printer: Lehigh Press, Inc.

5 6

Library of Congress Cataloging in Publication Data

Davis, Dale.
    How to quickly and accurately master ECG interpretation.

    Bibliography: p.
    Includes index.
    1. Electrocardiography.   2. Heart—Diseases—Diagnosis.
I. Title. [DNLM: 1. Electrocardiography. WG 140 D261h]
RC683.5.E5D33   1985   616.1'207547   84-28923
ISBN 0-397-50665-1

PREFACE

How to Quickly and Accurately Master ECG Interpretation is designed as an easy yet comprehensive approach to basic ECG interpretation. What has been available to the student in the past was either a book that was much too elementary with no reference value, or a complicated ECG manual that was difficult to complete without extra help. This book is a mixture of both methods, combined into one easy-to-understand program that can be used not only for quick and comprehensive learning, but also as a reference and a study guide.

Chapters 1 through 9 cover the fundamental knowledge necessary to evaluate normal 12-lead ECGs; and Chapters 10 through 15 cover the specialized criteria necessary to interpret abnormal 12-lead ECGs.

The book is presented in a simply organized step-by-step learning process, and includes easy-to-understand diagrams that enhance the text and assure comprehension of the electrophysiology of the normal and abnormal ECG, rather than just memorization of criteria. I have intentionally chosen simplicity in favor of exactness in some areas of the book in order to make learning uncomplicated.

A summary of each ECG abnormality discussed in a particular chapter is presented on a two-page display at the end of the chapter and is divided into three parts:

1. A diagram of the heart demonstrates the ECG abnormality, with the ECG leads necessary for examination placed around the heart in their correct positions.
2. Criteria necessary for recognition of the abnormality are listed directly below the heart diagram.
3. A 12-lead ECG that is representative of the ECG abnormality is displayed on the opposite page, with the previously designated leads observed around the heart diagram and in the criteria section tinted in blue for final correlation.

Practice ECGs with answers comprised of interpretations that relate only to the topic discussed in the chapter are included at the end of each ECG abnormality chapter. These ECGs are designed to reinforce the one concept just learned, without the student having to concern himself with other abnormalities.

The arrhythmia chapter is an introduction to basic arrhythmias rather than an exhaustive study on the subject. Each arrhythmia is presented with a diagram of the electrical conduction system with the respective abnormality depicted, a list of criteria for recognition, and at least one representation of the arrhythmia.

The last chapter includes ECGs and answers consisting of interpretations of assorted abnormalities. These are to be interpreted by the student after completing the book, since the student will now be able to make differential diagnoses using all the knowledge gained.

This book is directed toward the student in the allied health, nursing, or medical fields who desires the ability to interpret both routine and abnormal ECGs. Reading the text and interpreting the ECGs at the end of each chapter and at the end of the book will enable the reader to interpret ECGs skillfully and rapidly, and to understand the electrophysiology of normal and abnormal ECG patterns.

Dale Davis, RCT

CONTENTS

How to Quickly
and Accurately Master
ECG Interpretation

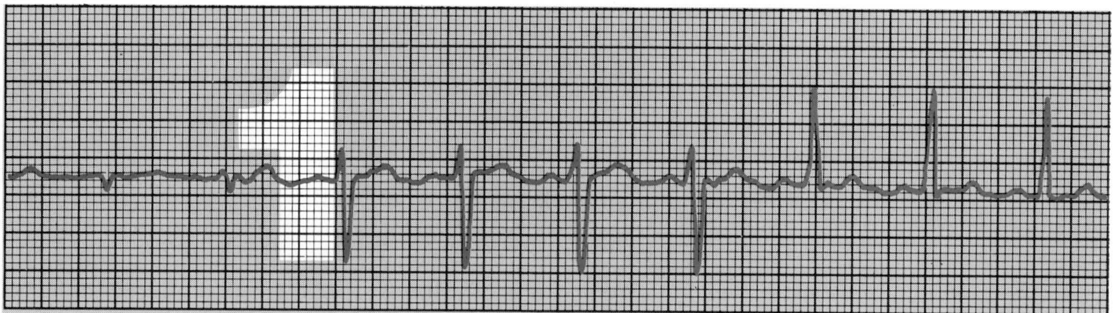

What Is an Electrocardiogram?

An electrocardiogram (ECG) is a recording of the electrical activity occurring in the heart each time it contracts.

Electrodes are placed on designated areas of the patient's body, and by the use of various combinations of these electrodes, twelve different views of the same electrical activity are demonstrated on the ECG graph paper. Each separate view of the heart is called an *ECG lead.* In routine testing we use a twelve-lead ECG, consisting of three standard leads and three augmented leads that view the heart in the frontal plane, and six precordial or chest leads that view the heart in the horizontal plane.

Electrodes are placed on both the wrists and on the left ankle of the patient to obtain the standard and augmented leads, but the electrodes actually may be placed anywhere on the respective limbs or upper and lower torso, and the same view of the heart is recorded. A fourth electrode is placed on the right ankle to stabilize the ECG, but this electrode takes no part in lead formation.

STANDARD AND AUGMENTED LEAD PLACEMENT

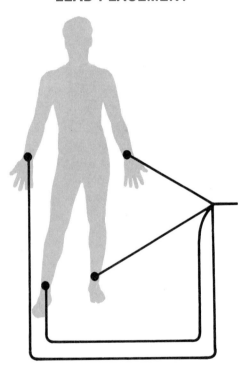

HOW TO QUICKLY AND ACCURATELY MASTER ECG INTERPRETATION

STANDARD LEADS

The standard leads are called *bipolar leads* because they are composed of two electrodes—one that is negative and one that is positive—and the ECG records the difference in electrical potential between them.

LEAD I

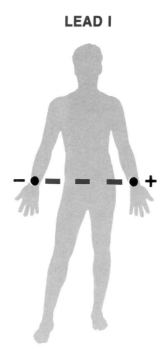

Lead I is composed of the right arm, which is designated as negative, and the left arm, which is considered positive.

LEAD II

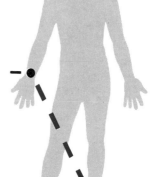

Lead II is composed of the right arm, which is made negative, and the left leg, which is considered positive.

WHAT IS AN ELECTROCARDIOGRAM?

Lead III is made up of the left arm, which is designated as negative, and the left leg, which is considered positive.

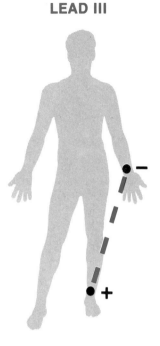

The three standard leads form a triangle over the body and have a mathematical relationship to one another as described by Einthoven: The height or depth of the recordings in lead I plus lead III equals the height or depth of the recordings in lead II.

EINTHOVEN'S TRIANGLE

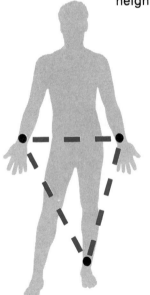

II   =   I   +   III

HOW TO QUICKLY AND ACCURATELY MASTER ECG INTERPRETATION

AUGMENTED LEADS

The same three electrodes used in the standard leads—left arm, right arm, and left leg—are used for augmented lead composition, only in different combinations. The augmented leads are considered unipolar leads because they comprise one positive electrode—either the left arm, right arm, or left leg—recording the electrical potential at that one point with reference to the other two remaining leads. Because of the manner in which these leads are arranged, the voltage is extremely low and must be augmented in order to equal the voltage of the remainder of the ECG. This increase is accomplished by the ECG machine.

LEAD AVR

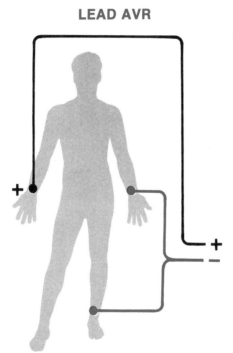

AVR—Augmented voltage of the right arm
The right arm is the positive electrode in reference to the left arm and left leg. This lead records the electrical activity of the heart from the direction of the right arm.

LEAD AVL

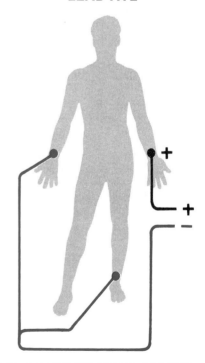

AVL—Augmented voltage of the left arm
The left arm is the positive electrode in reference to the right arm and the left leg. This lead views the electrical activity of the heart from the direction of the left arm.

WHAT IS AN ELECTROCARDIOGRAM?

AVF—Augmented voltage of the left foot

The left foot or the left leg is the positive electrode in reference to the left arm and the right arm. This lead sees the electrical activity of the heart from the direction of the bottom of the heart.

LEAD AVF

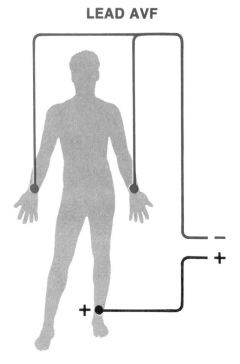

PRECORDIAL LEADS

The six precordial leads are unipolar leads and view the electrical activity of the heart in the horizontal plane. The following positions are used for placement of a suction cup lead on the chest in order to obtain the correct precordial lead placement:

PRECORDIAL LEAD PLACEMENT

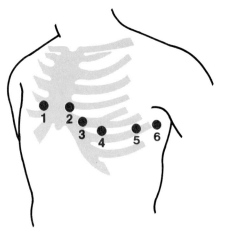

- V_1 4th intercostal (between the ribs) space immediately to the right of the sternum
- V_2 4th intercostal space immediately to the left of the sternum
- V_3 Directly between V_2 and V_4
- V_4 5th intercostal space—left midclavicular (mid-collarbone) line
- V_5 5th intercostal space—left anterior axillary (armpit) line
- V_6 5th intercostal space—left midaxillary line

HOW TO QUICKLY AND ACCURATELY MASTER ECG INTERPRETATION

The precordial leads view the heart in the horizontal plane. Imagine sawing the body into two parts at the level of the heart and lifting off the top part of the body and looking down at the heart.

PRECORDIAL LEADS VIEW THE HEART IN THE HORIZONTAL PLANE

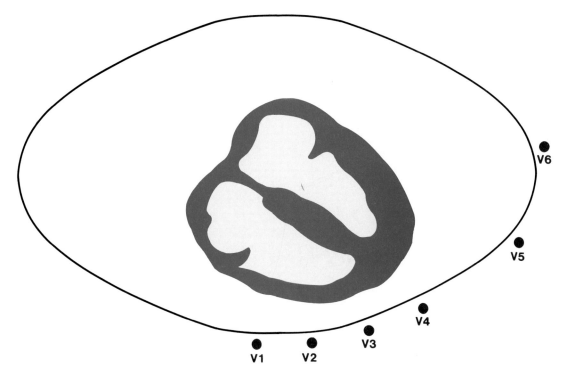

V_1 and V_2 are placed over the right ventricle.
V_3 and V_4 lie over the interventricular septum.
V_5 and V_6 are placed over the left ventricle.

Cardiac Cells

DEPOLARIZATION AND REPOLARIZATION

Each cardiac cell is surrounded by and filled with a solution that contains ions. The three ions that we will be concerned with are sodium (Na^+), potassium (K^+), and calcium (Ca^{++}). In the resting period of the cell, the inside of the cell membrane is considered negatively charged and the outside of the cell membrane is positively charged. The movement of these ions inside and across the cell membrane constitutes a flow of electricity that generates the signals on an ECG.

When an electrical impulse is initiated in the heart, the inside of a cardiac cell rapidly becomes positive in relation to the outside of the cell. The electrical impulse causing this excited state and this change of polarity is called *depolarization.* An electrical impulse begins at one end of a cardiac cell, and this wave of depolarization propagates through the cell to the opposite end. The return of the stimulated cardiac cell to its resting state is called *repolarization.* This phase of recovery allows the inside of the cell membrane to return to its normal negativity. Repolarization begins at the end of the cell that was just depolarized. The resting state is maintained until the arrival of the next wave of depolarization.

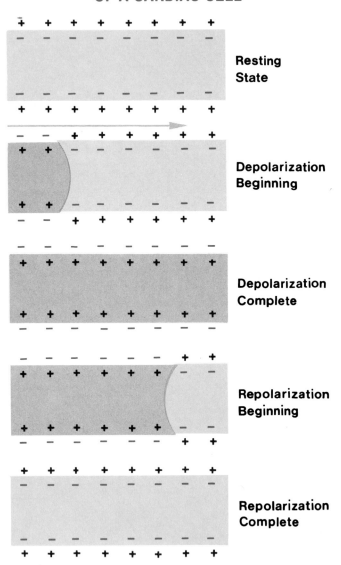

DEPOLARIZATION AND REPOLARIZATION
OF A CARDIAC CELL

Resting
State

Depolarization
Beginning

Depolarization
Complete

Repolarization
Beginning

Repolarization
Complete

Once the cardiac cells have been depolarized, a second wave of depolarization cannot occur until the first depolarization is completely finished. This is called the *absolute refractory period.* Immediately following this, the *relative refractory period* occurs during repolarization, at which time the cardiac cell is capable of being depolarized again but only by a strong stimulus.

ELECTROPHYSIOLOGIC PROPERTIES OF A CARDIAC CELL

Automaticity. The heart can begin and maintain rhythmic activity without the aid of the nervous system. A heart removed from the body has the ability to beat on its own for a period of time. The highest degree of automaticity is found in the pacemaker cells of the sinus node. The atria, atrioventricular (AV) node, bundle of His, bundle branches, Purkinje fibers, and the ventricular myocardium have a lesser degree of automaticity.

Excitability. A cardiac cell will respond to an electrical stimulus with an abrupt change in its electrical potential. Each cardiac cell that receives an electrical impulse will change its ionic composition and its respective polarity. Once an electrical potential begins in a cardiac cell it will continue until the entire cell is polarized.

Conductivity. A cardiac cell transfers an impulse to a neighboring cell very rapidly, so that all areas of the heart appear to depolarize at once. This principle is the same as that which applies to the electrical wiring on Christmas tree lights: The electrical wire propagates the electrical impulse to each light in succession in such a short span of time that all of the lights appear to light together. The velocity of transfer varies in the different cardiac tissues:

200 mm/second in the AV node
400 mm/second in ventricular muscle
1000 mm/second in atrial muscle
4000 mm/second in the Purkinje fibers

VELOCITY OF CONDUCTION OF ELECTRICAL IMPULSES

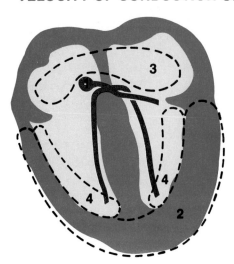

1. 200 mm/second
2. 400 mm/second
3. 1000 mm/second
4. 4000 mm/second

CARDIAC CELLS

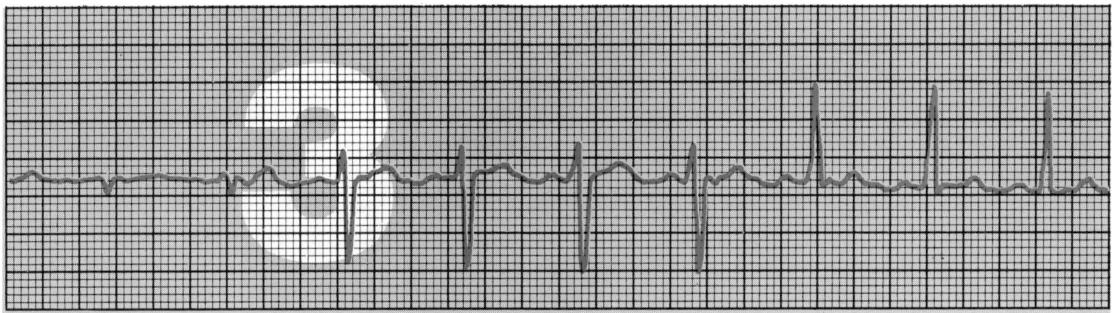

Anatomy
of the Heart
and the Electrical
Conduction System

ANATOMY

The heart is a muscular organ whose ultimate purpose is to pump blood to all the tissues of the body and thus to nourish them with oxygen. This is accomplished with a four-compartment heart. The two smaller upper chambers are the receiving chambers, called the *left atrium* and *right atrium,* and are divided by a wall called the *interatrial septum.* The two lower chambers, called the *ventricles,* are divided by a thicker wall, called the *interventricular septum.* The ventricles are responsible for pumping blood out of the heart. The right ventricle pumps unoxygenated blood a very short distance to the lungs, and the left ventricle has the more demanding job of pumping oxygenated blood throughout the entire circulatory system. Therefore, the left ventricular walls must be thicker than those of the right. The walls of the heart are composed of three distinct layers: (1) the endocardium, which is the thin membrane lining the inside of the cardiac muscle; (2) the cardiac muscle, called the myocardium; and (3) the epicardium, which is a thin membrane lining the outside of the myocardium.

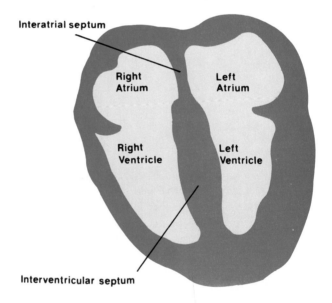

Interatrial septum

Right
Atrium

Left
Atrium

Right
Ventricle

Left
Ventricle

Interventricular septum

Unoxygenated blood is returned from the body to the right atrium. It flows into the right ventricle, where it is pumped a short distance into the lungs by way of the pulmonary artery to become oxygenated, and then is ready to be delivered back to the body. It begins its journey back by first entering the left atrium by way of the pulmonary veins. It then flows into the left ventricle and is pumped out to the entire body via the aorta to nourish the tissues with oxygen.

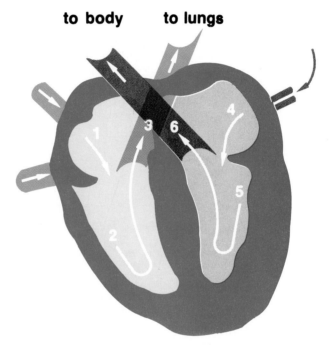

to body   **to lungs**

1. **Unoxygenated blood returns to the right atrium from the superior and inferior vena cava.**
2. **Blood proceeds to the right ventricle.**
3. **Blood is pumped into the pulmonary artery and into the lungs.**
4. **Oxygenated blood returns to the left atrium through pulmonary veins.**
5. **Blood flows to left ventricle.**
6. **Blood is pumped into the aorta and out to the body.**

Some terms referring to anatomical position will need to be understood in order to proceed with our description of the heart:

Anterior   Toward the front
Posterior   Toward the back
Inferior   Lower
Superior   Higher
Lateral   Toward the side
Apex   The pointed end of the ventricles

If we view the heart as it is seen lying within the chest, the right atrium and ventricle are in front of or lying anterior to the left atrium and ventricle. The left atrium and ventricle are in back of or lying posterior to the right atrium and ventricle. The atria are superior to the ventricles, and the ventricles are inferior to the atria.

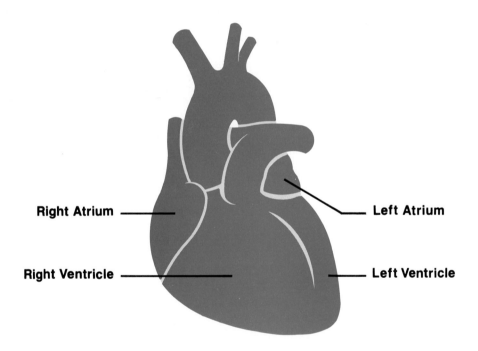

Right Atrium ——————   —————— **Left Atrium**

Right Ventricle ——————   —————— **Left Ventricle**

If we examine just the left ventricle as if we had removed it from the rest of the heart, we label the different walls of the chamber as anterior, posterior, inferior, and lateral.

HOW TO QUICKLY AND ACCURATELY MASTER ECG INTERPRETATION

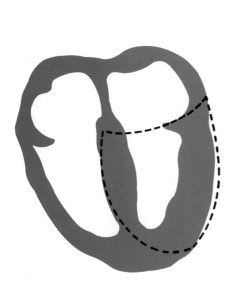 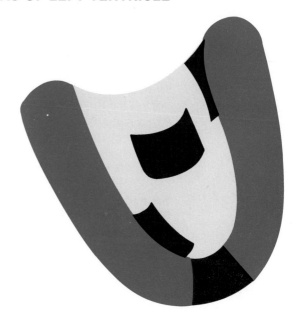

1. Anterior
2. Inferior
3. Posterior
4. Lateral

ELECTRICAL CONDUCTION SYSTEM

Now that you are familiar with the heart's function of pumping blood throughout the body, you should understand what actually initiates this mechanical action.

The electrical conduction system contains all the wiring and parts necessary to initiate and maintain rhythmic contraction of the heart. The system consists of (1) the sinoatrial (SA) node, (2) the internodal pathways, (3) the atrioventricular (AV) node, (4) the bundle of His, (5) the right bundle branch and the left bundle branch and its anterior and posterior divisions, and (7) the Purkinje fibers.

SA node. The cardiac impulse originates in the SA node, called "the pacemaker of the heart," located in the upper wall of the right atrium. The SA node has an elongated, oval shape and varies in size but is larger than the AV node.

SA NODE

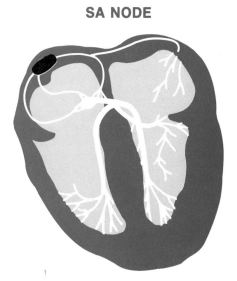

Internodal pathways. The cardiac impulse spreads through both atria by way of the internodal pathways and causes both atria to depolarize and then to contract.

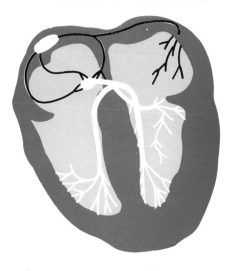

AV node. The depolarization wave arrives at the AV node, which is an oval structure approximately one third to one half the size of the SA node, and located on the right side of the interatrial septum; the wave is delayed there for approximately .10 second before arriving at the bundle of His.

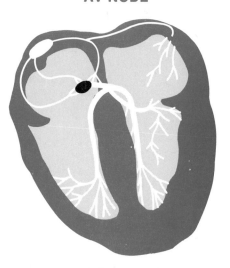

ANATOMY OF THE HEART AND THE ELECTRICAL CONDUCTION SYSTEM

Bundle of His. The cardiac impulse spreads to the thin bundle of threads connecting the AV node to the bundle branches, which are located in the right side of the interatrial septum just above the ventricles.

BUNDLE OF HIS

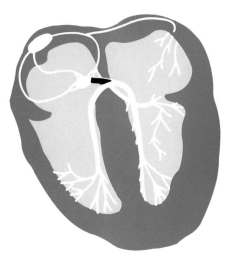

Right and left bundle branches. The right bundle branch is a slender fascicle that runs along the right side of the interventricular septum and supplies the electrical impulses to the right ventricle.

RIGHT BUNDLE BRANCH

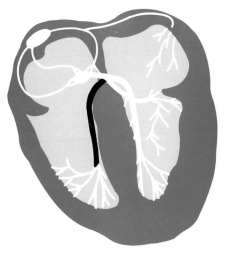

The left bundle branch is the other branch of the bundle of His and supplies electrical impulses to the left ventricle. It runs along the left side of the interventricular septum and divides almost immediately into an anterior and a posterior division.

The anterior fascicle supplies the anterior and superior portions of the left ventricle with electrical impulses.

LEFT ANTERIOR FASCICLE

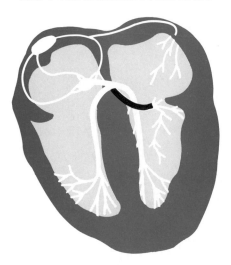

The posterior fascicle supplies the posterior and inferior portions of the left ventricle with electrical impulses.

LEFT POSTERIOR FASCICLE

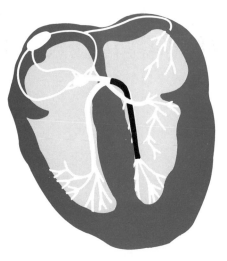

ANATOMY OF THE HEART AND THE ELECTRICAL CONDUCTION SYSTEM

Purkinje fibers. The bundle branches both terminate in a network of fibers that are located in both the left and right ventricular walls. The cardiac impulse travels into the Purkinje fibers and causes ventricular depolarization and then ventricular contraction.

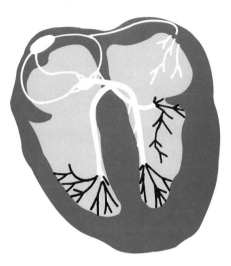

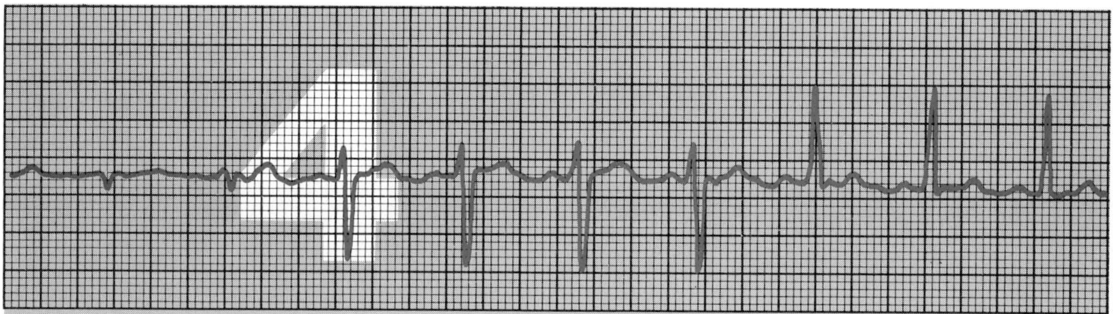

PQRSTU Waves, Complexes, Intervals, and Segments

The purpose of this chapter is to correlate the electrical events in the heart with the characteristic markings and configurations that occur during an ECG tracing.

WAVES AND COMPLEXES

A wave of depolarization begins in the SA node and spreads to both atria by way of the internodal pathways, and both atria depolarize. Atrial depolarization is represented by the P wave. P waves are usually upright and slightly rounded.

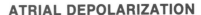

ATRIAL DEPOLARIZATION

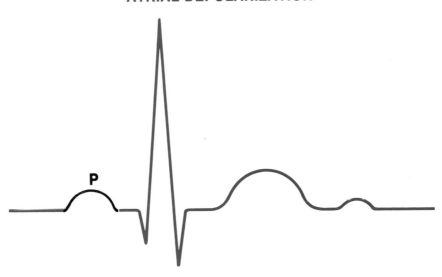

Remember, when cardiac cells depolarize they must also repolarize in order to regain their proper resting charge. Atrial repolarization is represented by the Ta wave, and its direction is opposite to that of the P wave. This wave is often not visible on the ECG because it usually coincides with the QRS complex and is impossible to recognize.

ATRIAL REPOLARIZATION

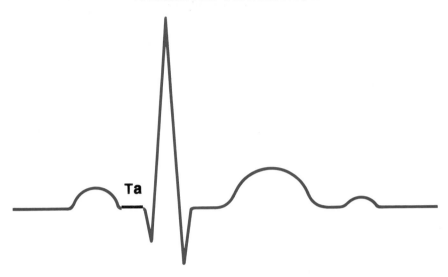

The wave of depolarization then spreads to the AV node, the bundle of His, the bundle branches, the Purkinje fibers, and the ventricular myocardium. Ventricular depolarization occurs and is represented by the QRS complex.

VENTRICULAR DEPOLARIZATION

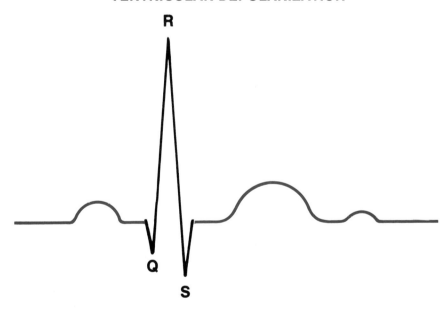

PQRSTU WAVES, COMPLEXES, INTERVALS, AND SEGMENTS

Ventricular repolarization is represented by the T wave. The T wave is normally upright and slightly rounded.

VENTRICULAR REPOLARIZATION

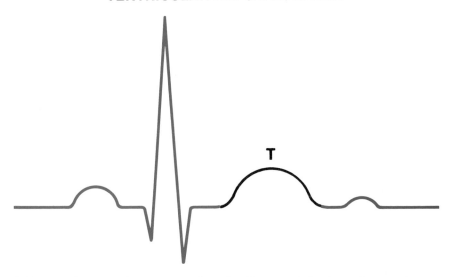

A U wave is sometimes seen after the T wave. It is thought to relate to the events of late repolarization of the ventricles. The U wave should be of the same direction as the T wave.

LATE REPOLARIZATION

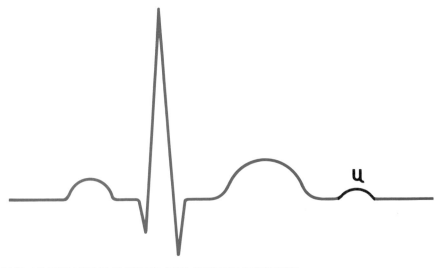

INTERVALS AND SEGMENTS

A point that helps in remembering the measurements we are going to discuss is that intervals contain waves, and that segments are the lines between the waves.

PR Interval. The time from the beginning of the P wave to the beginning of the QRS complex is called the *PR interval*. This time interval represents depolarization of the atria and the spread of the depolarization wave up to and including the AV node.

PR Segment. The PR segment represents the period of time between the P wave and the QRS complex.

ST Segment. The distance between the QRS complex and the T wave from the point where the QRS complex ends (J point) to the onset of the ascending limb of the T wave is called the *ST segment.* On the ECG, this segment is a sensitive indicator of myocardial ischemia or injury.

QT Interval. The time from the beginning of the QRS complex to the end of the T wave is called the *QT interval.* This interval represents both ventricular depolarization and repolarization.

Ventricular Activation Time. The time from the beginning of the QRS complex to the peak of the R wave is called the *ventricular activation time* and represents the time necessary for the depolarization wave to travel from the inner surface of the heart (endocardium) to the outer surface of the heart (epicardium).

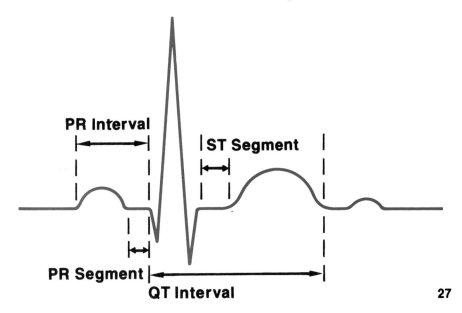

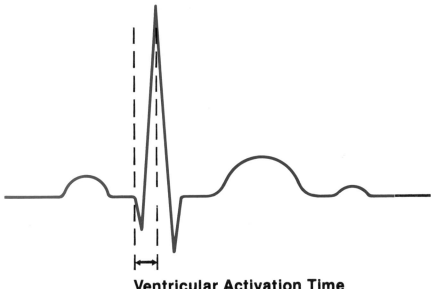

Ventricular Activation Time

KINDS OF QRS COMPLEXES

Our point of reference on the ECG is the isoelectric line. This is the flat line before the P wave or right after the T or U wave. Any stylus movement above this line is considered positive, and any stylus movement below this line is considered negative.

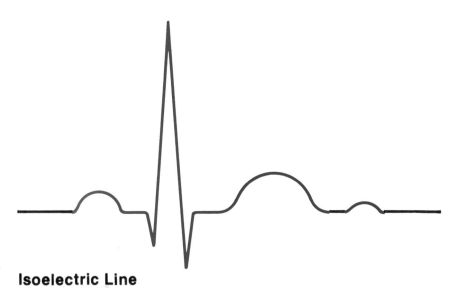

Isoelectric Line

A QRS complex may be composed of a Q wave, R wave, and an S wave, or various combinations thereof.

R wave is a positive deflection.
Q wave is a negative deflection before an R wave.
S wave is a negative deflection after an R wave.

R waves are only positive waves and Q and S waves are only negative waves. We always call a ventricular depolarization complex a QRS complex whether all three waves are present or not.

It is possible to have more than one positive wave in a QRS complex. These positive waves can only be R waves, and to differentiate between the two R waves the second R wave is labeled R prime (R'). The repetition of an S wave is designated by the use of S prime (S').

DIFFERENT KINDS OF QRS COMPLEXES

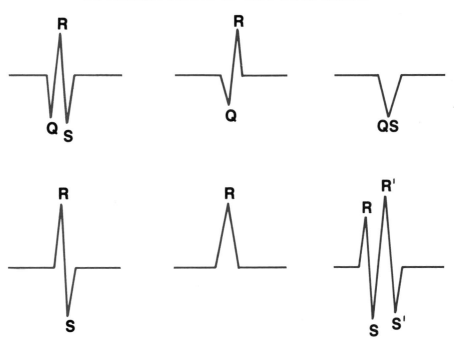

An R wave is a positive deflection.
A Q wave is a negative deflection before an R wave.
An S wave is a negative deflection after an R wave.

PQRSTU WAVES, COMPLEXES, INTERVALS, AND SEGMENTS

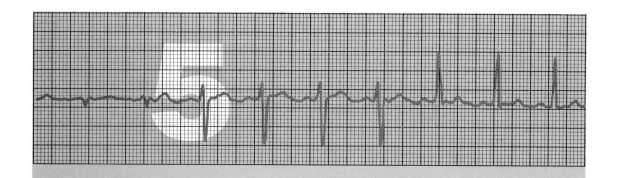

ECG Graph Paper
and Measurements

TIME AND VOLTAGE

Before understanding the important measurements of the PQRSTU complex, you should become familiar with the ECG graph paper.

On the vertical axis we measure voltage or height in millimeters (mm). Each small square is 1 mm high and each large square is 5 mm high. The isoelectric line is always our reference point.

VOLTAGE

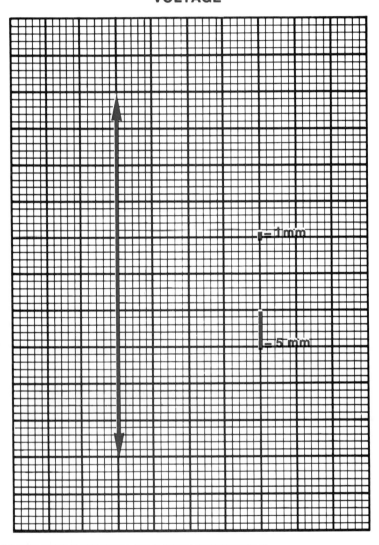

R waves are measured from the top of the isoelectric line to the top point of the R wave. Q and S waves are measured from the bottom of the isoelectric line to the bottom point of the Q or S wave. ST elevation is measured from the top of the isoelectric line to the ST segment, and ST depression is measured from the bottom of the isoelectric line to the ST segment.

VOLTAGE MEASUREMENTS

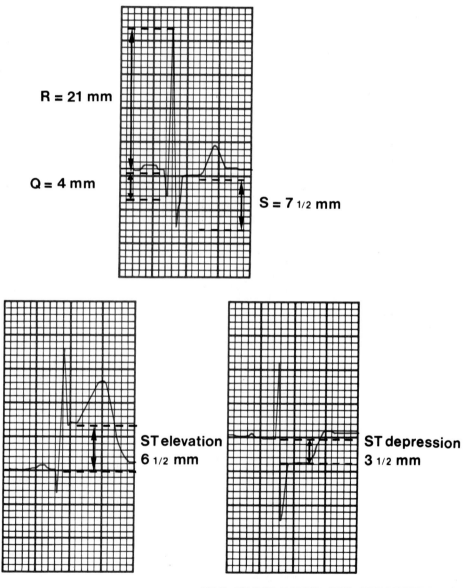

R = 21 mm

Q = 4 mm

S = 7 1/2 mm

ST elevation
6 1/2 mm

ST depression
3 1/2 mm

ECG GRAPH PAPER AND MEASUREMENTS

On the horizontal axis we measure time in seconds. Each small square is .04 second in duration and each large square is .20 second in duration. Five large squares = 1 second (5 × .20).

TIME IN SECONDS

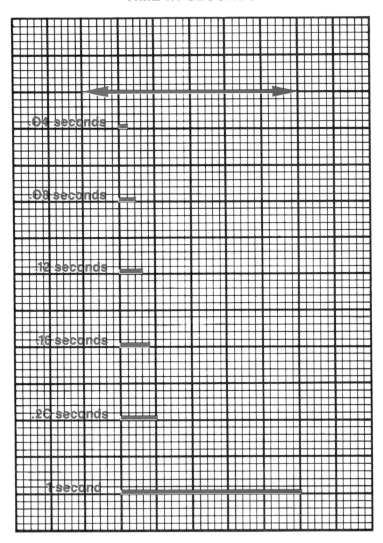

MEASUREMENTS

During our ECG analysis we will be measuring and examining the PR and QRS intervals.

PR interval. Atrial depolarization and AV conduction time are represented by the PR interval. Measure from the beginning of the P wave, where the P wave lifts off the isoelectric line, to the beginning of the first wave of the QRS complex. Count along the horizontal axis every .04 second (.04, .08, .12, .16, and .20, etc.) until you obtain the correct distance between the two points; this is the PR interval in seconds. The normal range for a PR interval is .12 to .20 second. If the rate of conduction of the sinus impulse through the AV node is faster than .12 second in duration, the term *accelerated conduction* is used. If the rate of conduction of the sinus impulse through the AV node is slower than .20 second, then *first degree AV block* is present.

PR MEASUREMENTS

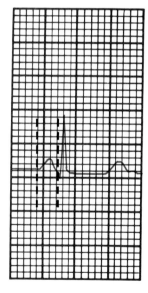

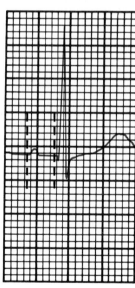

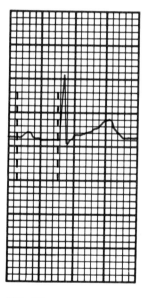

**PR .12
Accelerated
AV conduction**

PR .18

**PR .26
First degree
AV block**

ECG GRAPH PAPER AND MEASUREMENTS

QRS interval. Ventricular depolarization is represented by the QRS interval. Measure from the beginning of the first wave of the QRS where it lifts off the isoelectric line, to the end of the last wave of the QRS where it meets the isoelectric line. Count along the horizontal axis every .04 second until you obtain the distance between the two points; this is the QRS interval in seconds. The normal range for a QRS interval is .04 to .11 second.

QRS MEASUREMENTS

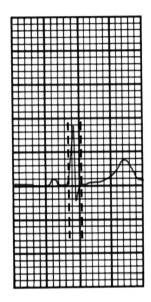

QRS .06

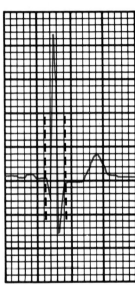

QRS .10

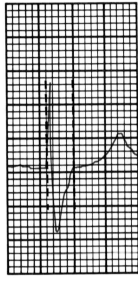

QRS .16

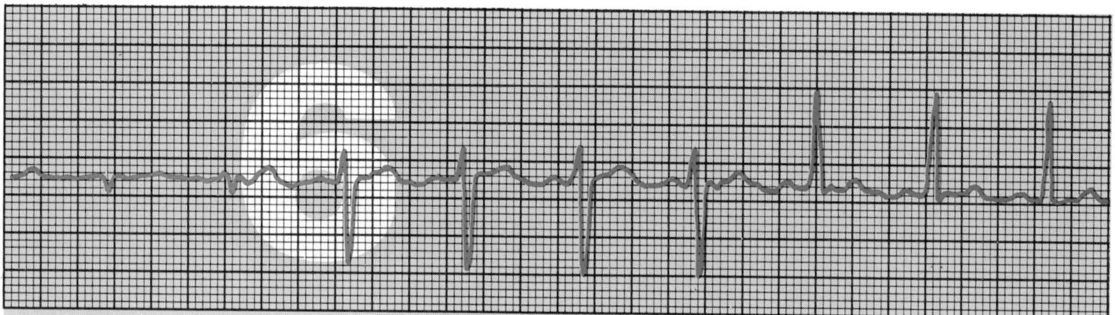

Determination of Heart Rate and Normal Heart Rhythms

DETERMINATION OF HEART RATE

Heart rate is the number of heartbeats occurring in one minute. On an ECG, the heart rate is measured from R wave to R wave to determine the ventricular rate, and P wave to P wave to determine the atrial rate. Remember, QRS complexes represent ventricular depolarizations and P waves represent atrial depolarizations. In the ECGs presented for interpretation in the following chapters, both the atrial and ventricular rates will be identical.

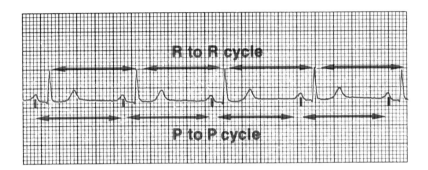

Two methods of calculating heart rate will be demonstrated:

1. **300-150-100-75-60-50.** This method is the easiest and quickest for rate determination. Choose an R wave that falls on or close to a heavy black line on the ECG paper. The first heavy black line to the right is the *300* line, the second is the *150* line, the third is the *100* line, the fourth is the *75* line, the fifth is the *60* line, and the sixth is the *50* line. If the next R wave falls on the fourth heavy black line to the right, the heart rate is 75 beats per minute.

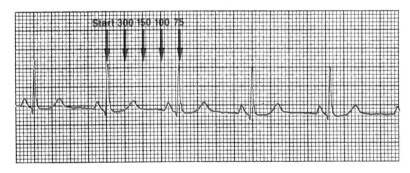

The heart rate is slightly above the rate of 75 beats per minute.

HOW TO QUICKLY AND ACCURATELY MASTER ECG INTERPRETATION

2. **Duration between R waves.** Count the duration in seconds between two R waves and divide this number into 60; this number is the heart rate.

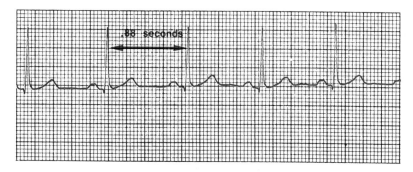

60 divided by .88 seconds = 68 beats per minute

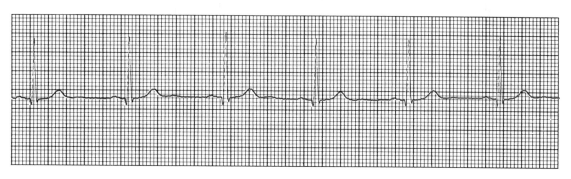

The heart rate is approximately 60 beats per minute.

SINUS RHYTHMS

A normal heart rhythm begins in the SA node and proceeds to depolarize the atria; then a P wave is inscribed on the ECG, representing atrial depolarization. The cardiac impulse travels to the AV node and the bundle of His, transverses the bundle branches and the Purkinje fibers, and a PR interval is recorded. The impulse then reaches the ventricular muscle and a QRS is displayed representing ventricular depolarization, which is followed by an isoelectric ST segment and a T wave representing ventricular repolarization. This heart rhythm is called *sinus rhythm*. The sinus rhythms are distinguished from one another by rate.

Sinus rhythm—60–100 beats per minute
Sinus bradycardia—below 60 beats per minute
Sinus tachycardia—above 100 beats per minute

CONDUCTION IN SINUS RHYTHM

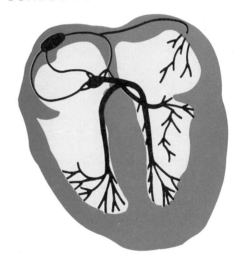

SINUS RHYTHMS

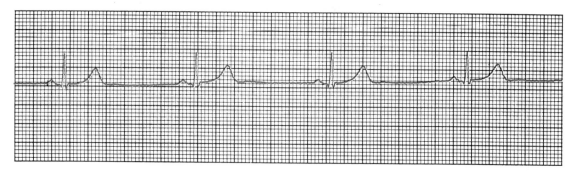

Sinus bradycardia at 43 beats per minute

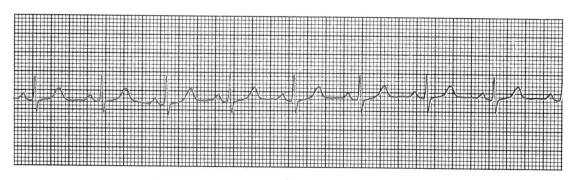

Sinus rhythm at 82 beats per minute

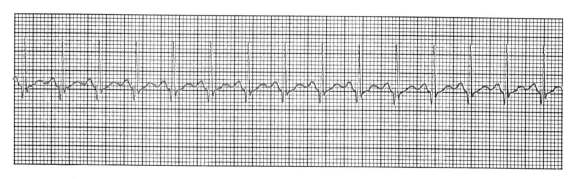

Sinus tachycardia at 149 beats per minute

DETERMINATION OF HEART RATE AND NORMAL HEART RHYTHMS

Sinus arrhythmia is a rhythm beginning in the SA node, and it demonstrates an irregular rate. The P-P and the R-R cycles vary more than .16 second.

SINUS ARRHYTHMIA

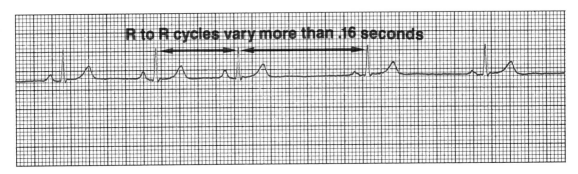

R to R cycles vary more than .16 seconds

RESPIRATORY SINUS ARRHYTHMIA

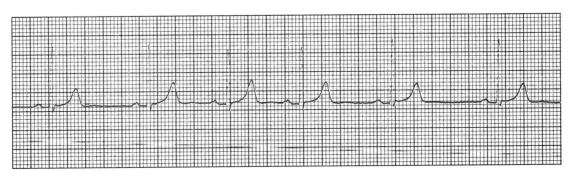

Heart rate increases with inspiration and decreases with expiration.

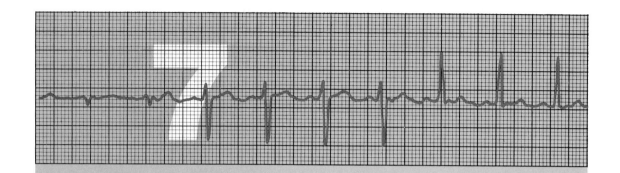

Normal 12-Lead ECG Configurations

VECTORS

Each of the 12 ECG leads views the heart from a different angle, so each ECG lead has a separate and sometimes distinct pattern. The standard and augmented leads view the heart in the frontal plane from six different positions, and the six precordial leads examine the heart in the horizontal plane. In order to demonstrate the configuration of each of the 12 ECG leads, we will show how the wave of depolarization travels within the heart by the use of a vector. A vector illustrates magnitude and direction of the depolarization waves within the heart. A mean QRS vector reveals an average of the depolarization waves in one portion of the heart (*e.g.*, the mean P vector representing atrial depolarization or the mean QRS vector denoting ventricular depolarization).

Let's review the electrical conduction system of the heart, consider the direction of depolarization within the atria and the ventricles, and label the system with vectors. The electrical impulse begins in the SA node and travels to both atria and depolarizes them. The initial wave of atrial depolarization spreads anteriorly through the right atrium and towards the AV node. The next waves of atrial depolarization travel posteriorly and toward the left atrium.

VECTORS

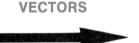

A vector points in the direction of depolarization.

ATRIAL DEPOLARIZATION

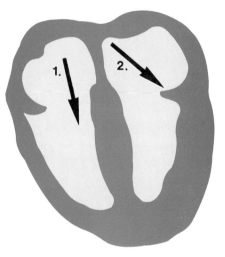

1. **Mean P vector for right atrium**
2. **Mean P vector for left atrium**

A mean P wave vector can be derived that represents the average direction and magnitude of depolarization through both atria. This will point downward and to the patient's left.

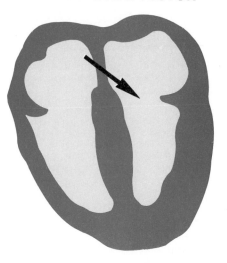

The mean P wave vector, which represents the average of right and left atrial depolarization, will point downward and to the patient's left.

A WAVE OF DEPOLARIZATION MOVING TOWARD AN ELECTRODE WILL RECORD A POSITIVE DEFLECTION ON AN ECG.

A WAVE OF DEPOLARIZATION TRAVELING AWAY FROM AN ELECTRODE WILL INSCRIBE A NEGATIVE DEFLECTION ON AN ECG.

A WAVE OF DEPOLARIZATION MOVING AT RIGHT ANGLES TO AN ELECTRODE WILL CAUSE EITHER NO DEFLECTION OR A VERY SMALL DEFLECTION ON AN ECG.

STANDARD, AUGMENTED, AND PRECORDIAL LEAD CONFIGURATIONS

The wave of atrial depolarization is moving downward and to the patient's left, directly toward lead II on an ECG. Lead II will record the tallest P wave. The wave of atrial depolarization is moving away from lead aVR so a negative P wave will be inscribed in this lead. The wave of atrial depolarization is moving at approximately right angles to lead III or aVL, so the smallest P wave will be seen in these leads.

MEAN P WAVE VECTOR

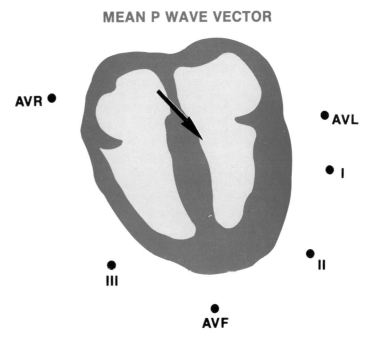

Lead II will have the tallest P wave because the mean P wave vector is moving directly toward it.

Lead aVR will have a negative P wave because the mean P wave vector is moving directly away from it.

Lead III or Lead aVL will have the smallest P wave because the mean P wave vector is moving at approximately right angles to it.

The P wave should always be positive in lead II and not wider than .11 second or taller than 2.4 mm. Lead aVR should always have an inverted P wave.

NORMAL P WAVE CONFIGURATIONS

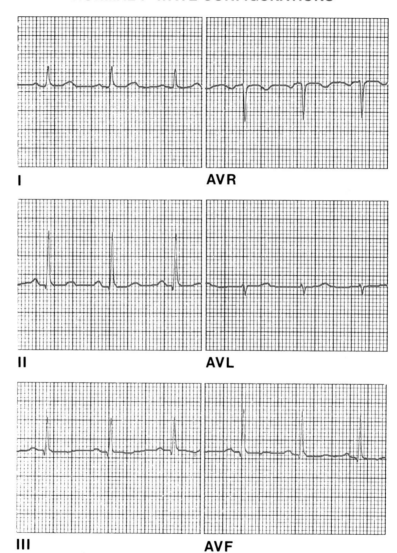

I   AVR

II   AVL

III   AVF

The P wave is most positive in II.
The P wave is negative in aVR.
The P wave is smallest in III or aVL.

NORMAL 12-LEAD ECG CONFIGURATIONS

After atrial depolarization the wave of depolarization travels to the ventricles by way of the AV node, bundle of His, and the bundle branches. We will divide ventricular depolarization into three main stages, each represented by a vector:

Vector 1. Septal activation and early right ventricular depolarization—the first activation in the ventricles occurs in the septum as it is depolarized from left to right. Early depolarization of the right ventricle also occurs.

VECTOR 1

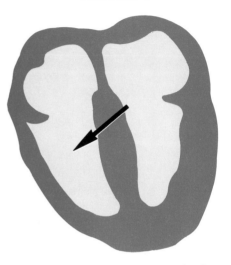

Septal and early right ventricular activation

Vector 2. Apical activation—the second major ventricular activation is the depolarization of the right and left ventricular apex and the completion of right ventricular depolarization.

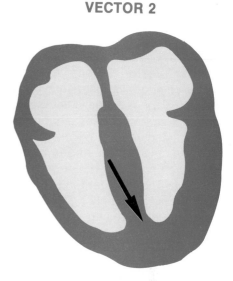

Apical activation

Vector 3. Left ventricular activation—the remainder of the left ventricle is depolarized toward the lateral wall. Because the right ventricle has already completed depolarization, the left ventricle will depolarize unopposed by the right, so large voltages will be inscribed at this time.

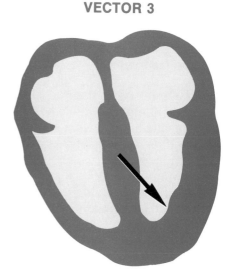

Left ventricular activation

NORMAL 12-LEAD ECG CONFIGURATIONS

If we place the six frontal and six precordial ECG leads on a diagram of the heart that depicts the three main stages of ventricular depolarization, you can easily see how each of the twelve ECG leads is derived. Vector 1, representing septal and early right ventricular activation, is moving away from all of the leads on the left side of the heart, so an initial negative deflection will be inscribed in the form of a Q wave. Leads on the right side of the heart will have the initial vector moving toward them, so an initial positive deflection will be recorded in the form of an R wave. The leads at the bottom of the heart that are at approximately right angles to the initial vector will demonstrate either no deflection or a very small deflection at this time.

Vector 2 represents the second major force of ventricular depolarization, labeled *apical activation,* and is moving approximately toward the ECG leads on the left side of the heart and at the bottom of the heart. A positive deflection in the form of an R wave will be recorded in the left heart leads, and because the vector is moving predominantly away from the right heart leads, a negative deflection or an S wave will be recorded.

Vector 3 illustrates the forces of left ventricular activation. The right ventricle has already depolarized, so the left ventricle will depolarize unopposed by the right and will display large positive voltages in the left heart leads as the electrical forces are moving toward them, and large negative voltages in the form of S waves in the right heart leads as the forces are moving away from them.

THE THREE STAGES OF VENTRICULAR DEPOLARIZATION

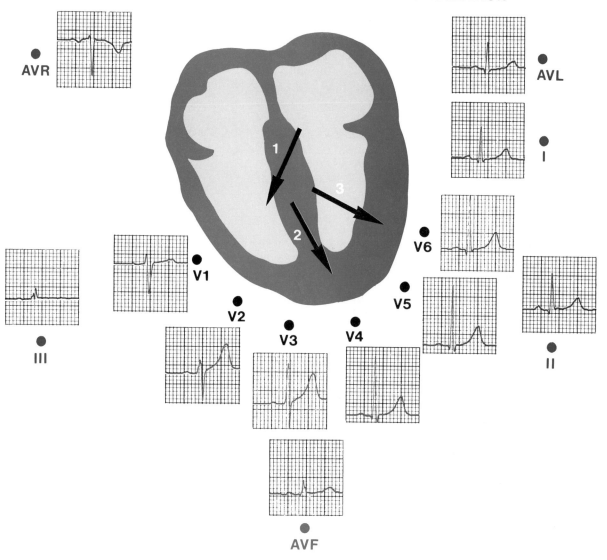

A wave of depolarization moving toward an electrode will record a positive deflection on an ECG.

A wave of depolarization traveling away from an electrode will inscribe a negative deflection on an ECG.

A wave of depolarization moving at right angles to an electrode will cause either no deflection or a very small deflection on an ECG.

NORMAL 12-LEAD ECG CONFIGURATIONS

Although the limb leads are open to some variability in their configuration, the chest leads must remain within a more standard format in order to be considered normal. The QRS should have a small R wave and a larger S wave in V_1, with the R wave becoming progressively larger and the S wave becoming progressively smaller or nonexistent when it reaches V_6. The area of transition where the R wave becomes equal to or larger than the S wave should occur in V_3 or V_4.

If the transition occurs in V_1 or V_2 it is considered an *early transition*, and if occurs in V_5 or V_6 it is considered a *late transition*.

PRECORDIAL LEAD CONFIGURATIONS

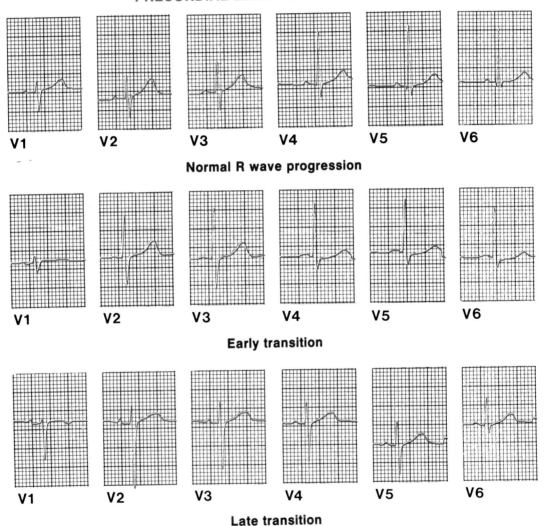

Normal R wave progression

Early transition

Late transition

HOW TO QUICKLY AND ACCURATELY MASTER ECG INTERPRETATION

A mean QRS vector can be derived that represents the average direction and magnitude of depolarization through both ventricles. This will point downward and to the patient's left, somewhere in the bottom quarter of the heart. Leads falling in this section of the heart will be predominantly positive because the mean QRS vector is moving toward them, and the leads falling outside this segment will have various combinations, depending upon their exact location.

MEAN QRS VECTOR

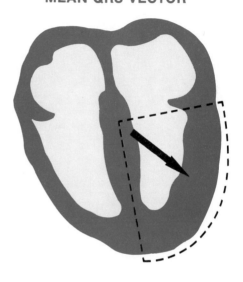

Ventricular repolarization is represented by the T wave and immediately follows ventricular depolarization. The T wave should be upright in leads I, II, aVL, aVF, and V_2–V_6; variable in leads III and V_1, and inverted in lead aVR. If a U wave is present it should be in the same direction as the T wave. The ST segment should be isoelectric, not varying more than 1 mm above or below the isoelectric line.

NORMAL T WAVE CONFIGURATIONS ON 12-LEAD ECG

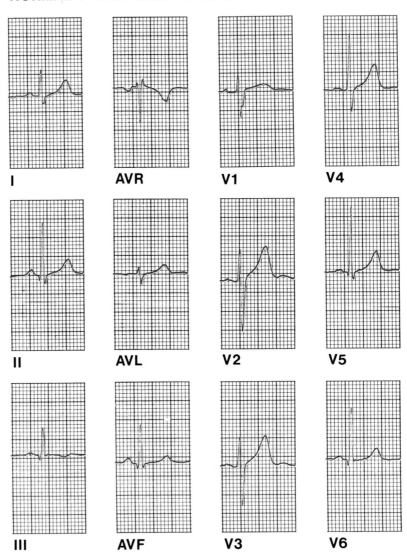

T waves should be upright in leads, I, II, aVL, aVF, V_2–V_6, and inverted in aVR. T waves are variable in leads III and V_1.

HOW TO QUICKLY AND ACCURATELY MASTER ECG INTERPRETATION

QRS Axis

HEXAXIAL REFERENCE SYSTEM

The QRS axis indicates the direction of the mean QRS vector within the heart. It refers to the average direction of depolarization that spreads through the ventricles. The QRS axis can be determined by using the hexaxial reference system. This system is formulated by placing the six frontal plane leads of an ECG around the heart in their respective ECG lead positions and by their positive poles. (See Chapter 1 if a review of this concept is needed.)

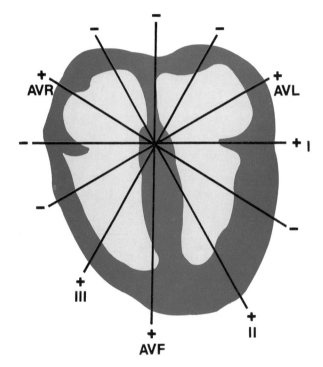

The six ECG limb leads are placed around the heart in their respective ECG lead positions by their positive poles.

The heart is divided, as if a circle, into segments each separated by 30°. Lead I's positive pole is at 0° and proceeding clockwise every division is at 30° increments in a positive category. Going in a counterclockwise direction from Lead I, every division is in 30° increments in a minus category.

HEXAXIAL REFERENCE SYSTEM

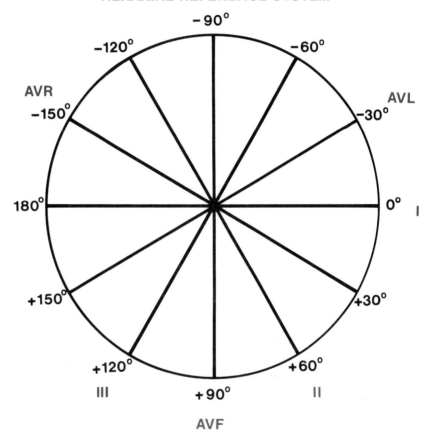

The axis is calculated using the hexaxial reference system.

A normal axis is from 0° to +90°. A left axis is from −1° to −90° and a right axis is from +91° to +180°. The last segment of the circle that is left undesignated is from −179° to −91°. This portion can be considered to be either extreme left or extreme right axis deviation.

AXIS

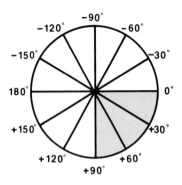

normal axis

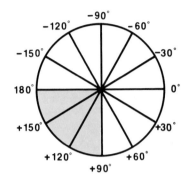

right axis

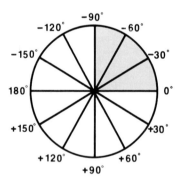

left axis

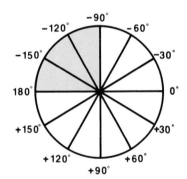

extreme right or left axis

AXIS DETERMINATION

There are three quick and easy ways to calculate the QRS axis on an ECG using leads I, II, III, aVR, aVL, and aVF:

1. The tallest QRS is found in the ECG lead that points directly toward the QRS axis.
2. The most negative QRS is seen in the ECG lead that points directly away from the QRS axis.
3. An equiphasic QRS (a positive and negative wave of the same voltage) is in the ECG lead that is at right angles to the QRS axis.

To begin axis determination, first look at the six frontal plane leads on your ECG and find the lead in which the QRS has the most voltage, either positive or negative. If the most voltage is positive (R wave), it points directly toward the axis. If the most voltage is negative (Q or S wave) it points directly away from the axis. If the most voltage is found in lead II and the voltage is positive, then the QRS axis will point directly toward that lead and the axis will be +60°. If the most voltage on an ECG is found in lead III, but the voltage is negative, then the QRS axis will point directly away from this lead and the axis will be −60°.

AXIS CALCULATIONS USING THE QRS COMPLEX WITH THE MOST VOLTAGE

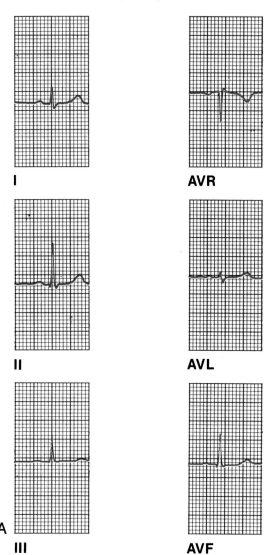

I   AVR

II   AVL

A
III   AVF

The QRS in lead II has the most voltage. The voltage is positive so the mean QRS vector is pointing directly toward lead II or at +60°. Axis = +60°.

QRS AXIS

AXIS CALCULATIONS USING THE QRS COMPLEX WITH THE MOST VOLTAGE

AXIS CALCULATIONS USING THE QRS COMPLEX WITH THE MOST VOLTAGE

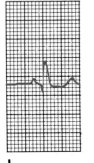

I

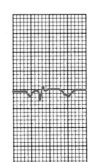

AVR

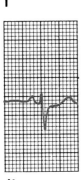

II

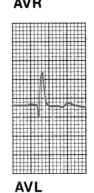

AVL

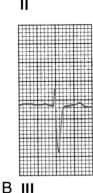

B III

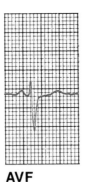

AVF

The QRS in lead III has the most voltage. The voltage is negative so the mean QRS vector is pointing directly away from lead III or at −60°. Axis = −60°.

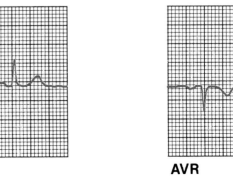

I

AVR

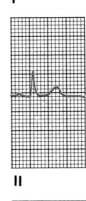

II

AVL

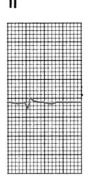

III

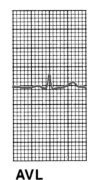

AVF

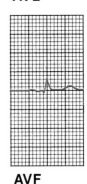

C

The QRS complexes in lead I and lead II have the most voltage. The voltage is equally positive in both leads so the mean QRS vector is pointing directly between lead I and lead II or at +30°. Axis = +30°.

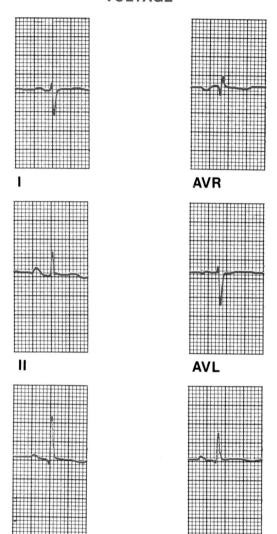

D III   AVF

The QRS in lead III has the most voltage. The voltage is positive so the mean QRS vector is pointing directly toward lead III or at +120°. Axis = +120°.

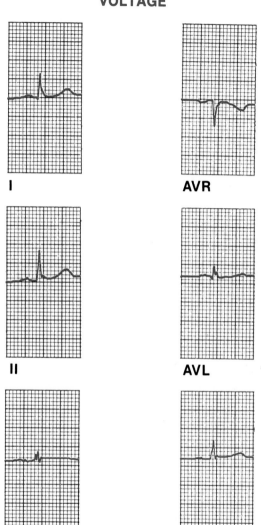

III   AVF   E

The QRS complexes in leads II and aVR have the most voltage. The voltage in aVR is negative so the mean QRS vector is pointing directly away from it or at +30°. The voltage in II is positive so the mean QRS vector is pointing directly toward it or at +60°. An average of the two voltages is +45°. Axis = +45°.

If you find an ECG that has an equiphasic QRS in a lead, then that lead is at right angles to the QRS axis. With an equiphasic QRS in lead I, your axis will be at right angles to lead I, either +90° or −90°. One more step is necessary in order to decide which direction to proceed in. Check lead II on the ECG. If that lead has a predominantly positive QRS, then the QRS axis is in that general direction, which would be +90°. If you check lead II and discover that the QRS is predominantly negative, then you know that the QRS axis is going away from lead II and that the axis would be −90°.

AXIS CALCULATIONS USING EQUIPHASIC QRS COMPLEXES

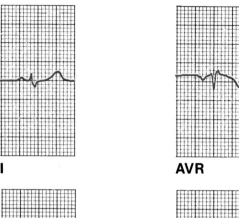

I

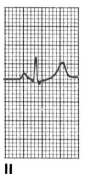

II

III

AVR

AVL

AVF

The axis is at right angles to the equiphasic QRS in lead I so the axis is either +90° or −90°. The QRS in lead II is positive, which indicates that the mean QRS vector is traveling in the general direction of +60°. Axis = +90°.

AXIS CALCULATIONS USING EQUIPHASIC QRS COMPLEXES

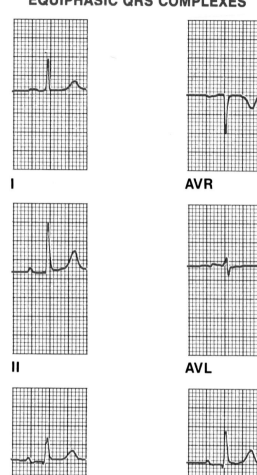

I

II

III

AVR

AVL

AVF

The axis is at a right angle to the equiphasic QRS in lead aVL so the axis is either +60° or −120°. The QRS in II is positive, which indicates that the mean QRS vector is traveling in the general direction of +60°. Axis = +60°.

QRS AXIS

AXIS CALCULATIONS USING EQUIPHASIC QRS COMPLEXES

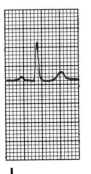

I

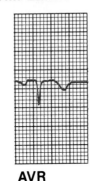

AVR

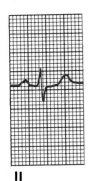

II

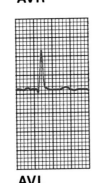

AVL

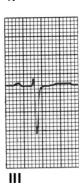

III

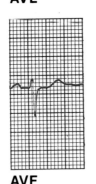

AVF

The axis is at right angles to the equiphasic QRS in lead II so the axis is either −30° or +150°. The QRS in III is negative, which indicates that the mean QRS vector is traveling away from +120°. Axis = −30°.

AXIS CALCULATIONS USING EQUIPHASIC QRS COMPLEXES

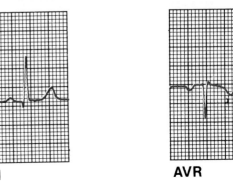

I

AVR

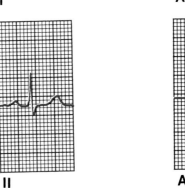

II

AVL

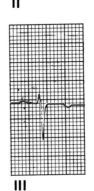

III

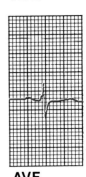

AVF

The axis is at right angles to the equiphasic QRS in lead aVF. The axis is either ±180 or 0°. The QRS in II is positive, which indicates that the mean QRS vector is traveling in the general direction of +60°. Axis = 0°.

HOW TO QUICKLY AND ACCURATELY MASTER ECG INTERPRETATION

Occasionally, you will find an ECG in which all of the six frontal plane leads are equiphasic. This arrangement makes it impossible to decide on a correct axis, and so we'll call this an indeterminate axis.

INDETERMINATE AXIS

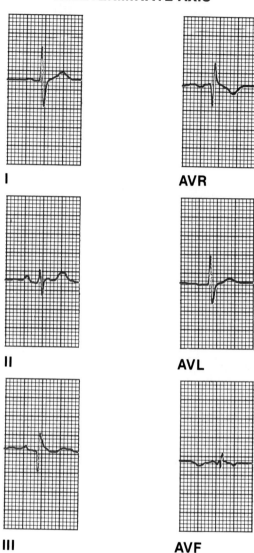

I

AVR

II

AVL

III

AVF

All QRS complexes are equiphasic, which makes axis calculations impossible.

QRS AXIS

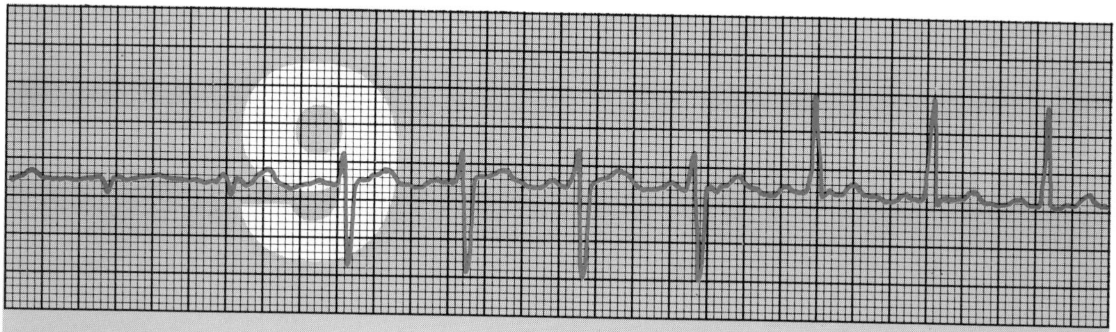

12-Lead ECG Interpretation

TECHNICALLY ACCURATE ECG TRACING

The most important part of ECG interpretation is to begin with a technically accurate tracing. Let's insure that the ECG has been recorded correctly. Using Einthoven's equation (lead II = lead I + lead III), the voltage in lead II should equal the voltage of both I and III together. The P wave should be positive in lead II and negative in aVR.

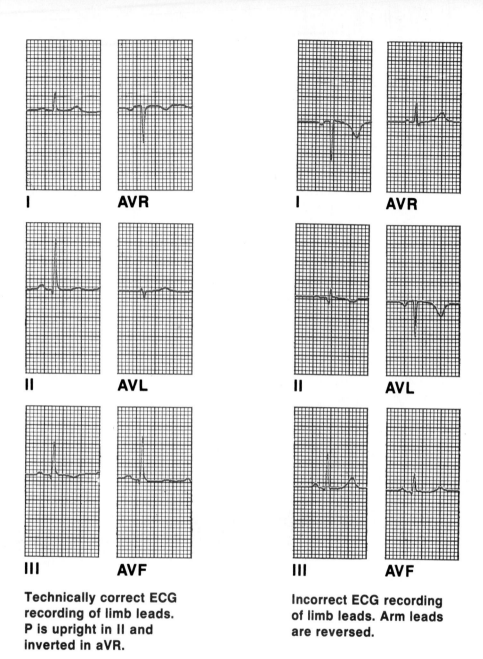

I   AVR   I   AVR

II   AVL   II   AVL

III   AVF   III   AVF

Technically correct ECG
recording of limb leads.
P is upright in II and
inverted in aVR.

Incorrect ECG recording
of limb leads. Arm leads
are reversed.

12-LEAD ECG INTERPRETATION

In the chest leads, normal R wave progression should be present. The R wave should be small in V_1 and should become progressively larger as it travels to V_6.

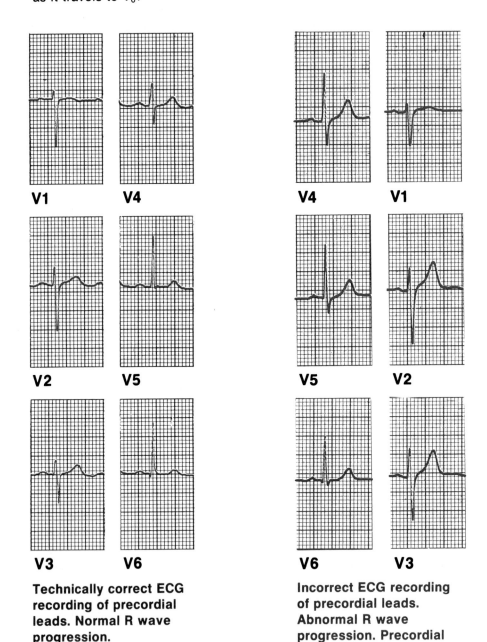

V1 **V4**

V2 **V5**

V3 **V6**

Technically correct ECG recording of precordial leads. Normal R wave progression.

V4 **V1**

V5 **V2**

V6 **V3**

Incorrect ECG recording of precordial leads. Abnormal R wave progression. Precordial leads interchanged.

ARTIFACT

Once we're assured of a technically correct ECG recording we now become concerned with the quality of the tracing. We're looking for an ECG recording that has no outside interference introduced into it and in which the lines making up the waves and intervals are satisfactory. Any outside markings on the ECG represent artifact. The three different types of artifact that are usually encountered are: (1) AC interference, (2) somatic muscle tremor, and (3) wandering baseline.

AC interference.   This artifact originates outside the patient and comes from electrical interference at the patient's bedside.

AC INTERFERENCE

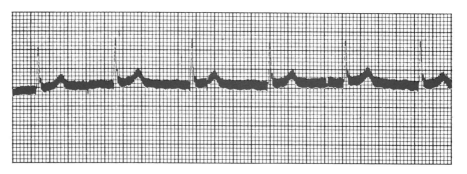

Somatic muscle tremor.   This artifact is created by the patient himself and usually involves tense muscles or muscle movement.

SOMATIC MUSCLE TREMOR

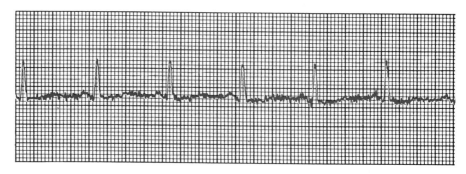

12-LEAD ECG INTERPRETATION

Wandering baseline. This is caused by poor electrode contact with the patient's skin. Dirty electrodes or insufficient electrode cream can inhibit good contact. The patient's skin may be oily, dirty, scaly, or have an excess amount of body hair, making good electrode contact impossible.

WANDERING BASELINE

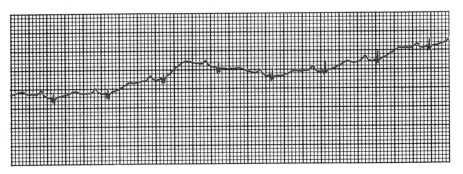

Any one of these artifacts makes the measurement of intervals and assessment of segments and waves extremely difficult, if not impossible.

12-LEAD ECG INTERPRETATION

Now that we have completed all the basic concepts of ECG interpretation, let's put them all together and form a guide to follow for all ECGs that require interpretation in the following chapters:

1. Measure the PR interval in lead II. A normal range is from .12 to .20 second. A PR interval shorter than .12 second is considered accelerated AV conduction, and a PR interval longer than .20 second is first degree AV block.
2. Measure the QRS interval in lead II. The normal range is from .04 to .11 second.
3. Calculate the QRS axis. A normal axis is from 0° to +90°. An axis from −1° to −90° is considered left axis deviation and an axis from +91° to +180° is a right axis deviation. An axis from −91° to −179° is either extreme left or right axis deviation.
4. Examine the ST segment for more than 1 mm of elevation or depression.
5. Check the T waves, which should be upright in all leads except aVR, V_1, and possibly III.
6. The heart rhythm will always be sinus rhythm.
7. If no abnormalities are present the interpretation will simply be sinus rhythm.

Each ECG record demonstrated in this chapter will conform with the following format for interpretation:

PR:
QRS:
QRS Axis:
Interpretation:

PR: .14

QRS: .08

QRS Axis: 75°

Interpretation: normal ECG

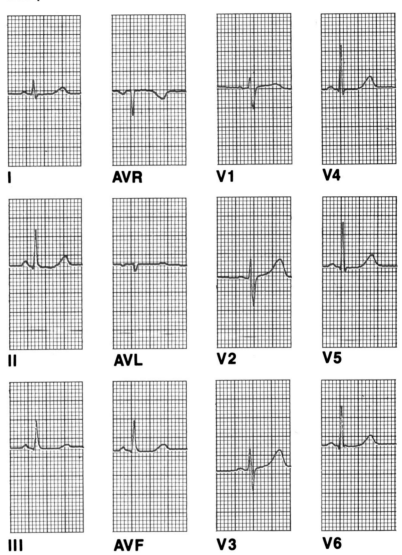

I   AVR   V1   V4

II   AVL   V2   V5

III   AVF   V3   V6

PR: .19

QRS: .08

QRS Axis: 0°

Interpretation: normal ECG

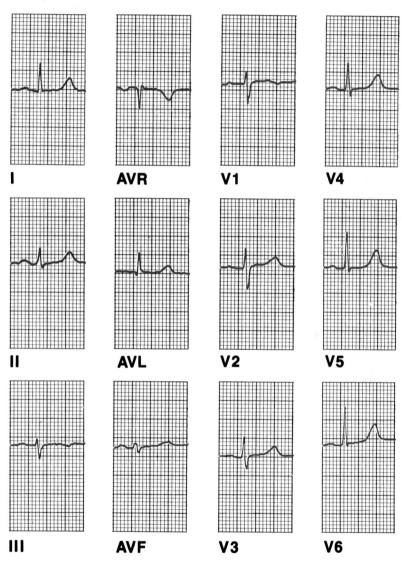

I AVR V1 V4

II AVL V2 V5

III AVF V3 V6

12-LEAD ECG INTERPRETATION

PRACTICE ECG 1

PR:

QRS:

QRS axis:

Interpretation

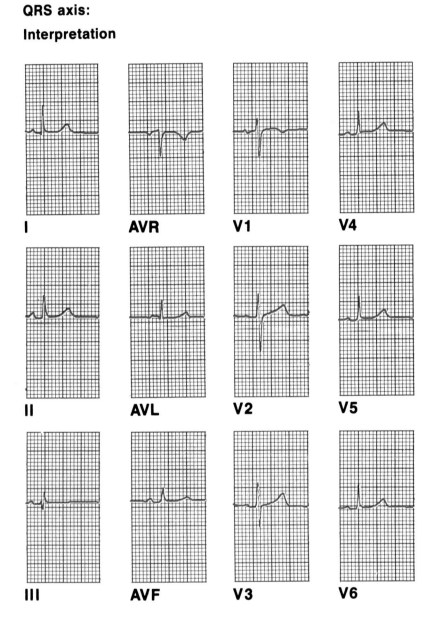

PRACTICE ECG 2

PR:

QRS:

QRS axis:

Interpretation:

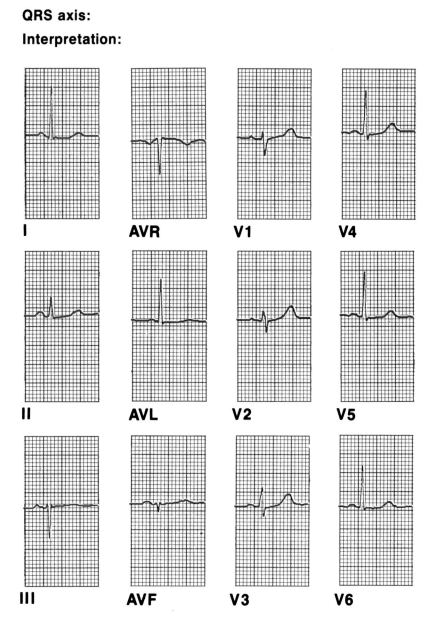

PRACTICE ECG 3

PR:

QRS:

QRS axis:

Interpretation:

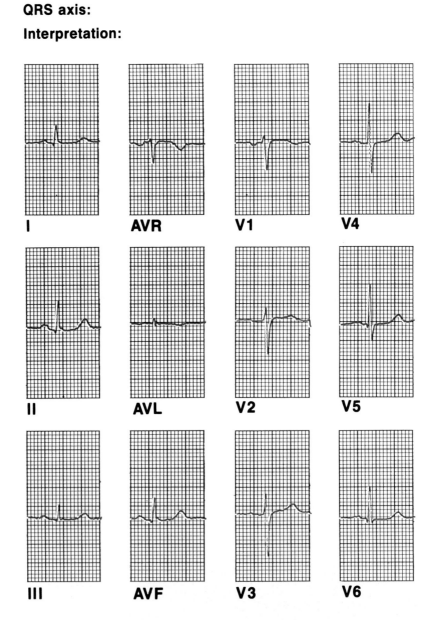

PRACTICE ECG 4

PR:

QRS:

QRS axis:

Interpretation:

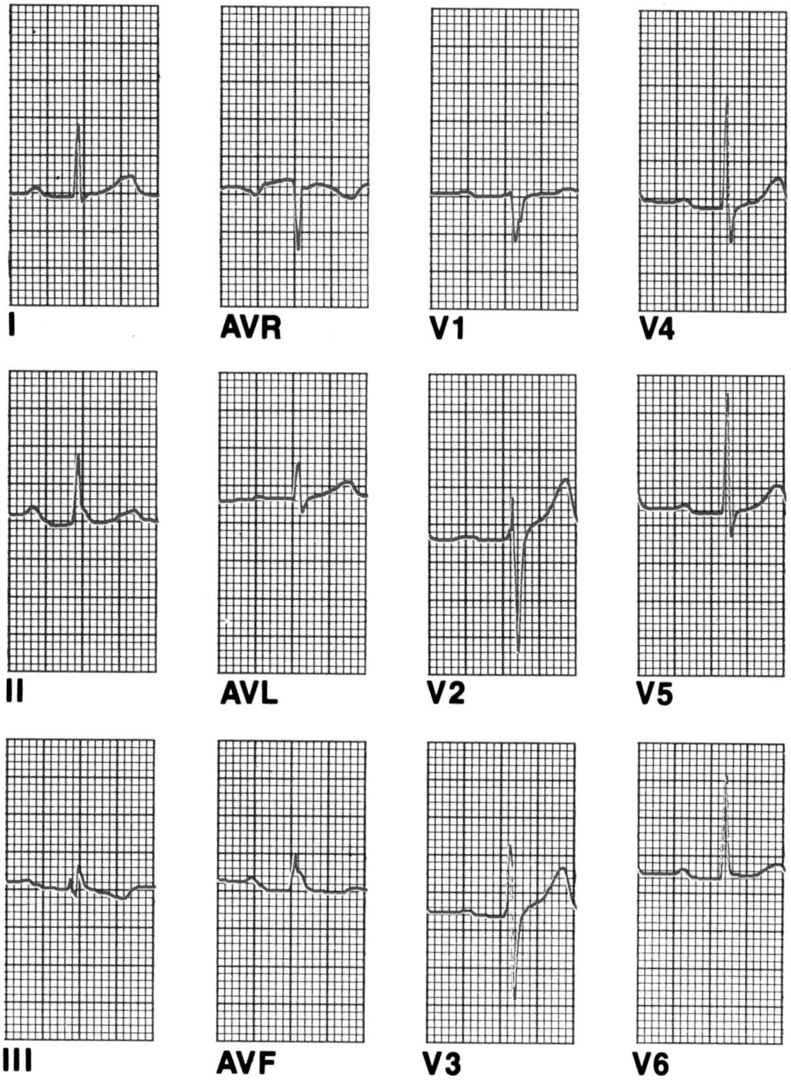

I AVR V1 V4

II AVL V2 V5

III AVF V3 V6

PRACTICE ECG 5

PR:

QRS:

QRS axis:

Interpretation:

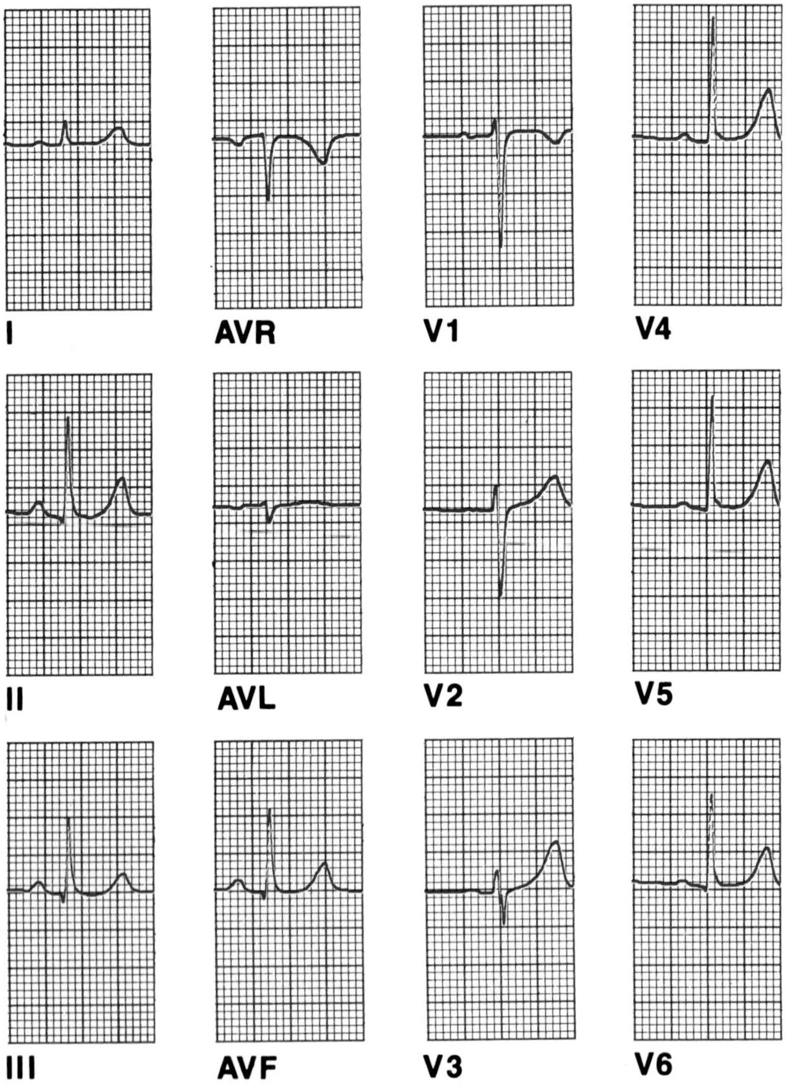

I	AVR	V1	V4
II	AVL	V2	V5
III	AVF	V3	V6

PRACTICE ECG 6

PR:

QRS:

QRS axis:

Interpretation:

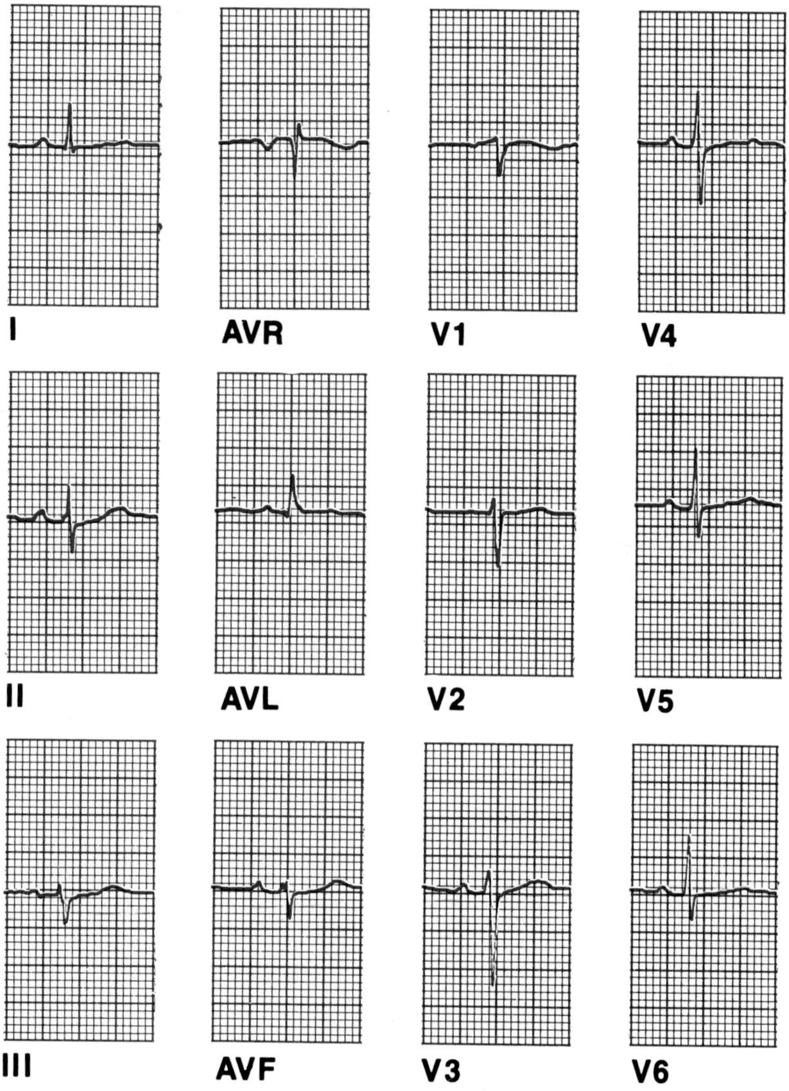

I AVR V1 V4

II AVL V2 V5

III AVF V3 V6

PRACTICE ECG 7

PR:

QRS:

QRS axis:

Interpretation:

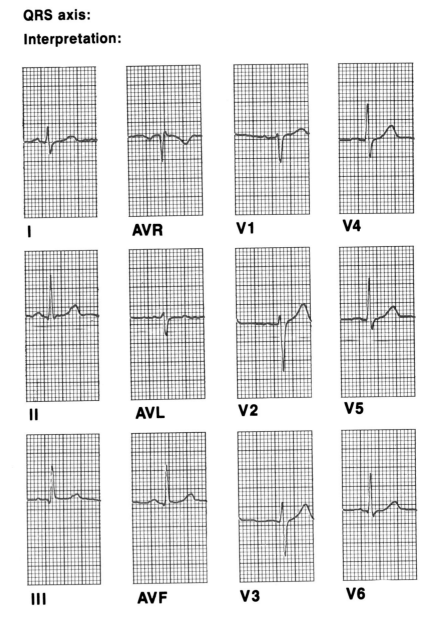

HOW TO QUICKLY AND ACCURATELY MASTER ECG INTERPRETATION

PRACTICE ECG 8

PR:

QRS:

QRS axis:

Interpretation:

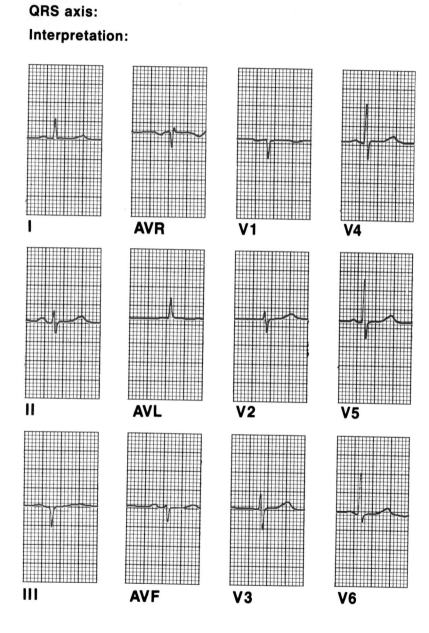

PRACTICE ECG 9

PR:

QRS:

QRS axis:

Interpretation:

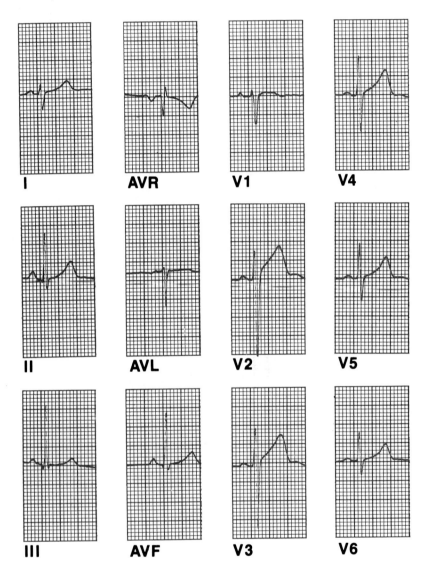

PRACTICE ECG 10

PR:

QRS:

QRS axis:

Interpretation:

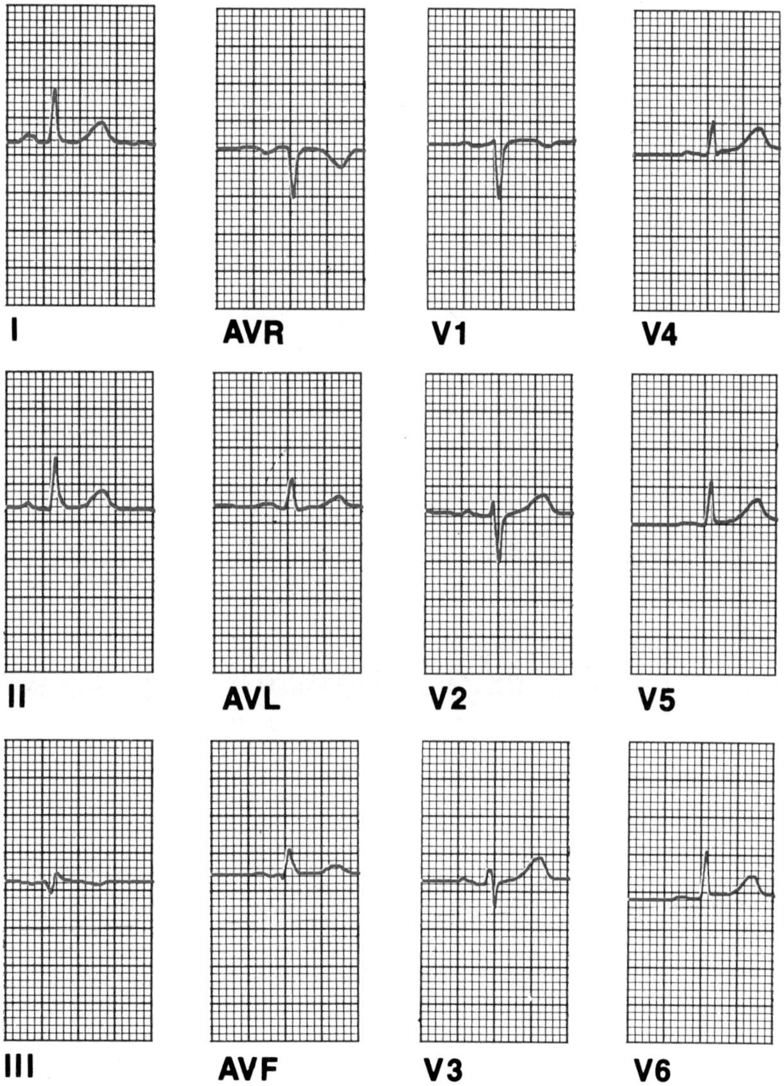

I	AVR	V1	V4
II	AVL	V2	V5
III	AVF	V3	V6

12-LEAD ECG INTERPRETATION

PR:

QRS:

QRS axis:

Interpretation:

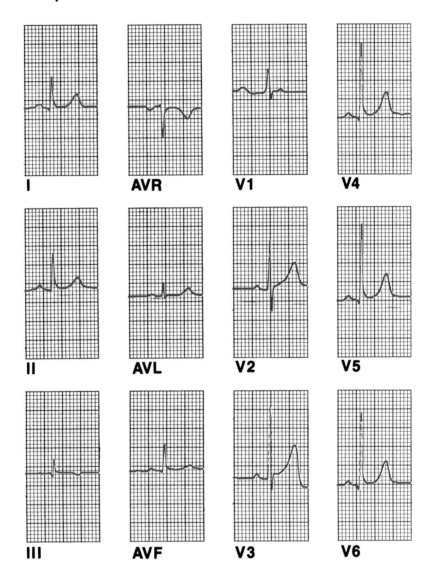

I AVR V1 V4

II AVL V2 V5

III AVF V3 V6

PRACTICE ECG 12

PR:

QRS:

QRS axis:

Interpretation:

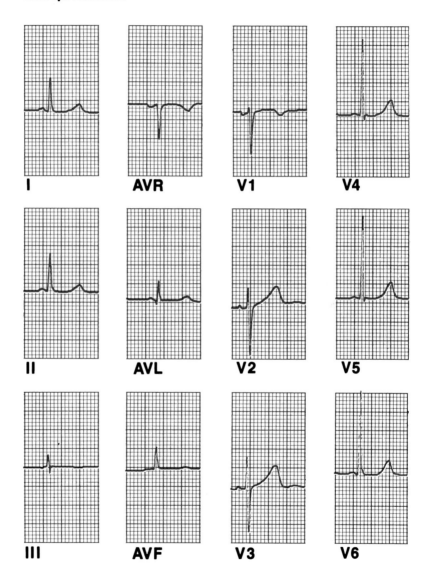

PRACTICE ECG 13

PR:

QRS:

QRS axis:

Interpretation:

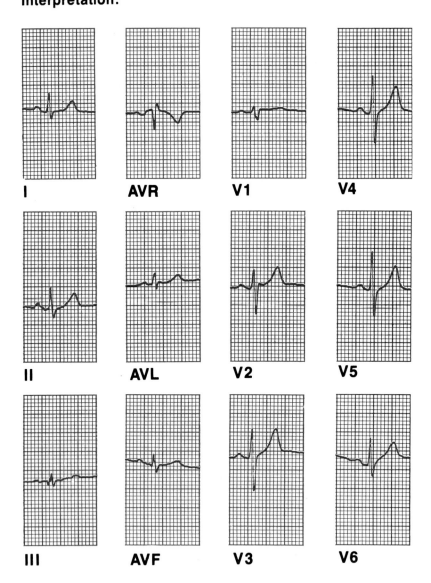

I	AVR	V1	V4
II	AVL	V2	V5
III	AVF	V3	V6

HOW TO QUICKLY AND ACCURATELY MASTER ECG INTERPRETATION

PRACTICE ECG 14

PR:

QRS:

QRS axis:

Interpretation:

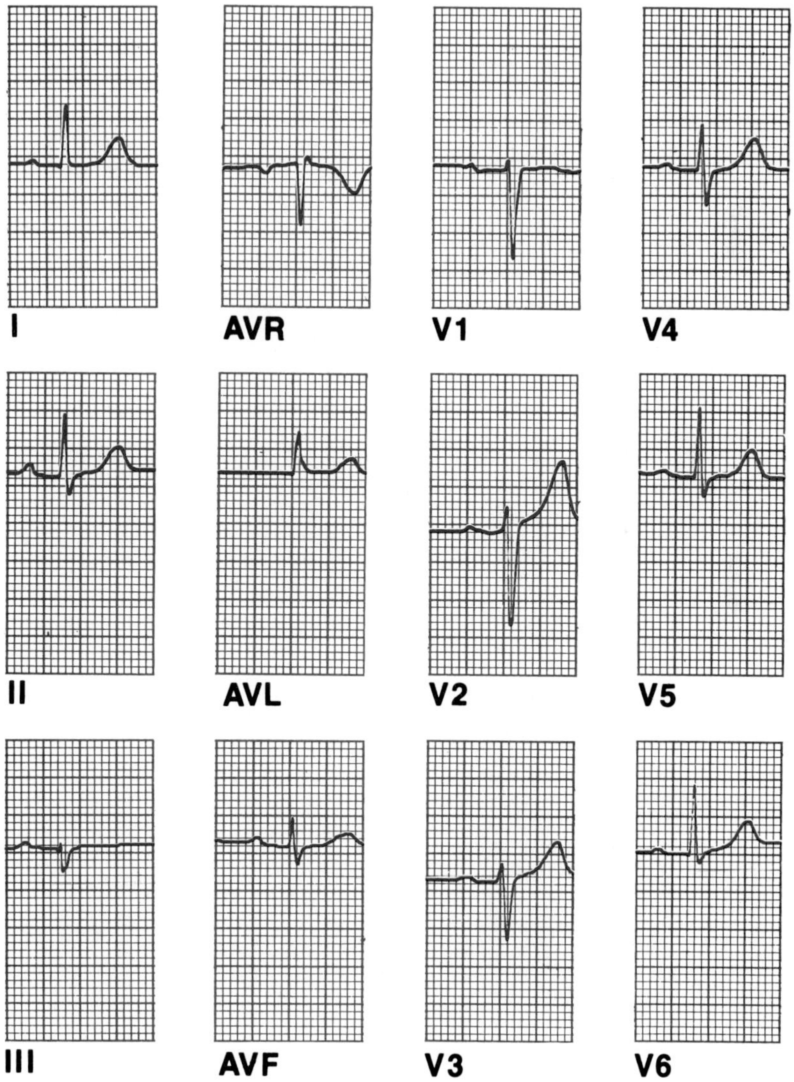

I AVR V1 V4

II AVL V2 V5

III AVF V3 V6

PRACTICE ECG 15

PR:

QRS:

QRS axis:

Interpretation:

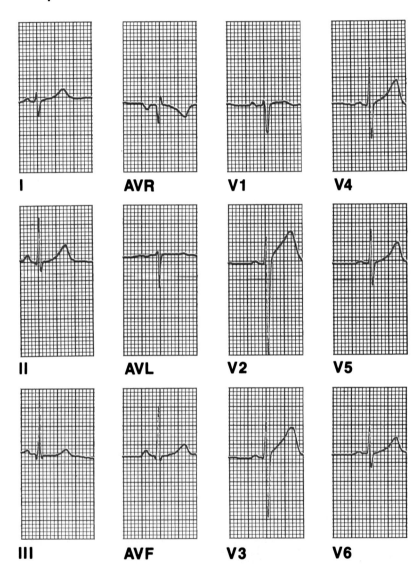

I AVR V1 V4

II AVL V2 V5

III AVF V3 V6

ANSWERS FOR PRACTICE ECGS

	PR	QRS	AXIS	INTERPRETATION
1.	.16	.06	+30°	Sinus rhythm
2.	.14	.07	0°	Sinus rhythm
3.	.16	.06	+60°	Sinus rhythm
4.	.26	.09	+30°	Sinus rhythm with first degree AV block
5.	.19	.08	+60°	Sinus rhythm
6.	.16	.07	−30°	Sinus rhythm with left axis deviation
7.	.16	.10	+90°	Sinus rhythm
8.	.16	.08	−30°	Sinus rhythm with left axis deviation
9.	.16	.08	+105°	Sinus rhythm with right axis deviation
10.	.18	.08	+30°	Sinus rhythm
11.	.15	.08	+30°	Sinus rhythm
12.	.10	.08	+45°	Sinus rhythm with accelerated AV conduction
13.	.16	.08	IND.	Sinus rhythm with indeterminate axis
14.	.22	.08	0°	Sinus rhythm with first degree AV block
15.	.14	.08	+110°	Sinus rhythm with right axis deviation

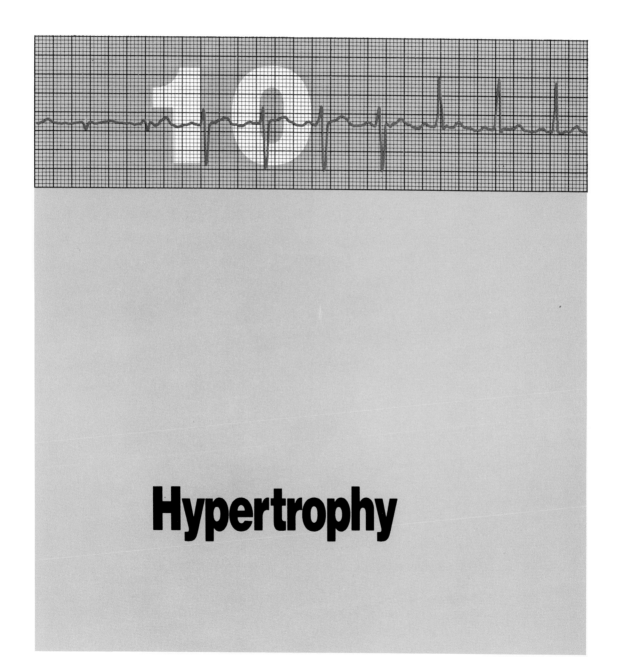

Hypertrophy

Hypertrophy is an increase in the thickness of the muscular wall of one of the chambers of the heart. Either or both of the atrial or ventricular walls can hypertrophy, and this is usually the result of a pressure or flow overload. Another term, which is often used interchangeably with *hypertrophy*, is *enlargement*.

ATRIAL

Left atrial hypertrophy. An increase in the size of the left atrial wall is called *left atrial hypertrophy*. The SA node initiates depolarization of the right atrium first, anteriorly and inferiorly towards the AV node, which we will label vector 1. Then the left atrium depolarizes in a posterior and leftward direction because it is located behind and to the left of the right atrium, and it is represented by vector 2.

NORMAL ATRIAL DEPOLARIZATION RECORDED IN V_1

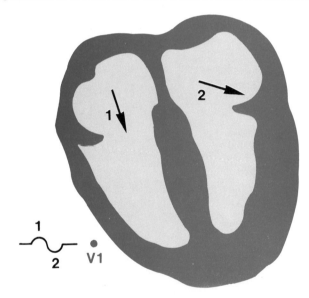

If we view atrial depolarization in lead V_1 on an ECG we will usually see a diaphasic P wave. The initial vector in the atria representing right atrial depolarization will be traveling toward V_1, and will inscribe an initial positive component of the P wave. The left atrial vector will be moving away from the V_1 electrode and will record a negative terminal portion of the P wave. If the left atrial wall is hypertrophied

HOW TO QUICKLY AND ACCURATELY MASTER ECG INTERPRETATION

there will be an increase in the amount of vectors traveling toward the left atrium, away from the V_1 electrode. This will cause the terminal portion of the P wave in V_1, representing left atrial depolarization, to enlarge to 1 mm or more deep.

ATRIAL DEPOLARIZATION

1. **Right atrial depolarization moving toward V_1 inscribes an initial positive deflection of the P wave.**
2. **Left atrial depolarization moving away from V_1 records a terminal negative deflection of the P wave.**

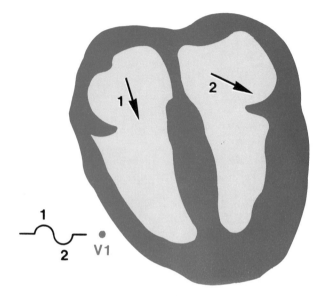

Normal Heart

1. **Right atrial depolarization moving toward V_1 inscribes an initial positive deflection of the P wave.**
2. **Depolarization of the enlarged left atrium moving away from V_1 produces a deeply inverted terminal portion of the P wave.**

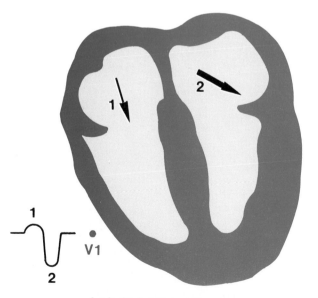

Left Atrial Hypertrophy

HYPERTROPHY

V₁ P WAVE CONFIGURATIONS

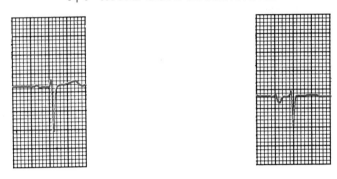

Normal   **Left Atrial Hypertrophy**

LEFT ATRIAL HYPERTROPHY

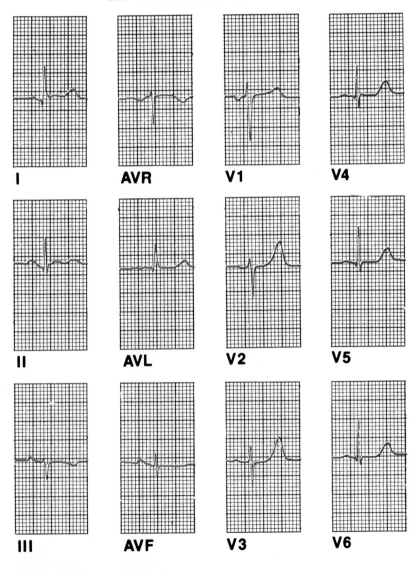

| I | AVR | V1 | V4 |

| II | AVL | V2 | V5 |

| III | AVF | V3 | V6 |

Right atrial hypertrophy. An increase in the size of the right atrial wall is called *right atrial hypertrophy.* If we use lead II to view atrial depolarization in a normal heart, we will notice an upright P wave not more than 2.4 mm high. The initial portion of atrial depolarization is represented by vector 1, which is traveling anteriorly and inferiorly toward lead II in a direct path, and which inscribes an upright deflection of the P wave. The second component of atrial depolarization is represented by vector 2, which is moving leftward and posteriorly, and only in the general direction of lead II; therefore it records a positive deflection of the P wave but with less voltage than vector 1.

NORMAL ATRIAL DEPOLARIZATION RECORDED IN LEAD II

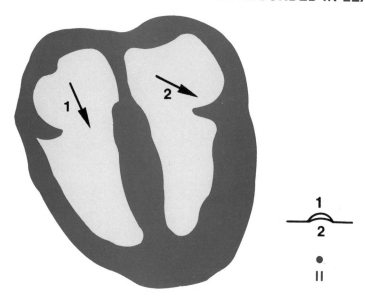

If the right atrium is hypertrophied there will be an increase in the amount of vectors traveling directly toward lead II, and a P wave higher than 2.4 mm will be recorded.

ATRIAL DEPOLARIZATION

1. Depolarization of the right atrium traveling toward II inscribes a positive deflection of the P wave.
2. Depolarization of the left atrium moving toward II records a positive deflection of the P wave.

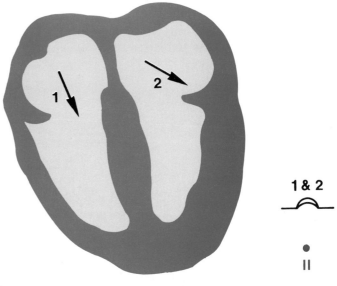

Normal Heart

1. Depolarization of the enlarged right atrium moving toward lead II inscribes a tall peaked P wave.
2. Depolarization of the left atrium moving toward lead II records a small upright P almost simultaneously with the right atrium.

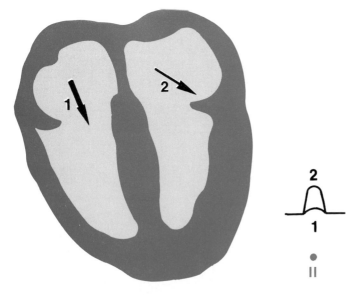

Right Atrial Hypertrophy

LEAD II P WAVE CONFIGURATIONS

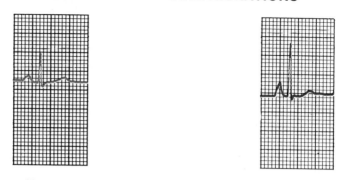

Normal   **Right Atrial Hypertrophy**

RIGHT ATRIAL HYPERTROPHY

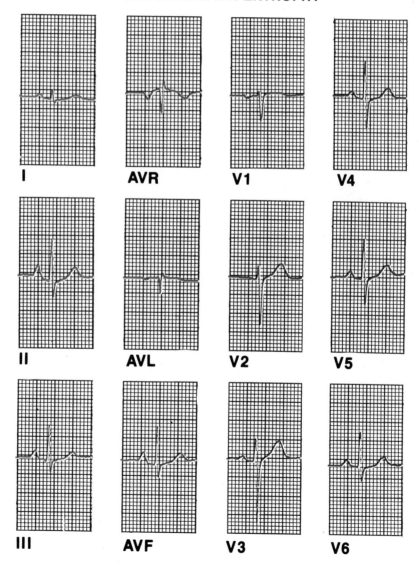

I	AVR	V1	V4
II	AVL	V2	V5
III	AVF	V3	V6

Biatrial hypertrophy. An enlargement of both the left and the right atria is called *biatrial hypertrophy.* The criteria for recognition are that of left and right atrial hypertrophy.

BIATRIAL HYPERTROPHY

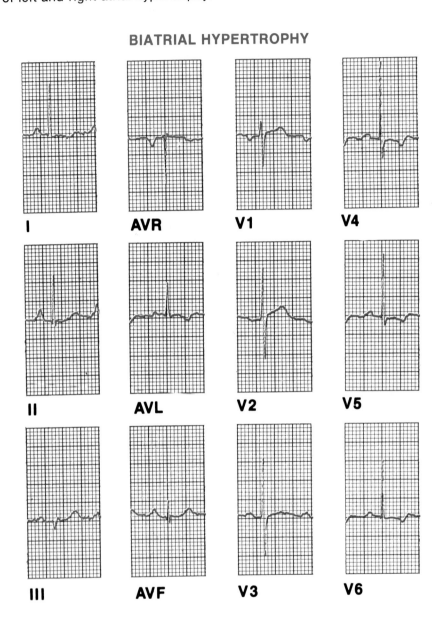

VENTRICULAR

The first stage of ventricular depolarization in the normal heart depicts septal activation and early right ventricular depolarization. V_1 will demonstrate a small R wave as depolarization travels toward it, and V_6 will show an initial small Q wave as depolarization proceeds away from it. The second stage of ventricular depolarization denotes apical activation. V_1 receives a negative deflection in the form of an S wave as depolarization moves away from it, and V_6 inscribes an R wave as depolarization is traveling toward it. In the last stage of ventricular depolarization, V_1 receives an increase in the size of the S wave while the main forces of depolarization, representing predominantly left ventricular depolarization, are moving away from it, and V_6 increases the R wave voltage as the wave of depolarization is moving toward it.

Left ventricular hypertrophy. An increase in the size of the wall of the left ventricle is called *left ventricular hypertrophy.* The left ventricular wall is approximately three times as thick as the right in a normal heart. When the wall of the left ventricle increases in thickness even more, large voltages are recorded in the leads over the hypertrophied left ventricle. Leads I, aVL, V_5, and V_6 will record the largest voltages in the form of tall R waves as the wave of depolarization moves toward them, and the right ventricular leads, V_1 and V_2, will increase their negative voltages as the wave of depolarization moves away from them. The increase in the muscle thickness of the ventricular walls increases the voltages over the hypertrophied area.

VENTRICULAR DEPOLARIZATION

The left ventricular wall is thicker than the right, causing the mean QRS vector to point leftward, rendering a large R wave in V_6 as the mean wave of depolarization moves toward the electrode, and recording a large S wave in V_1 as the mean wave of depolarization moves away from the electrode.

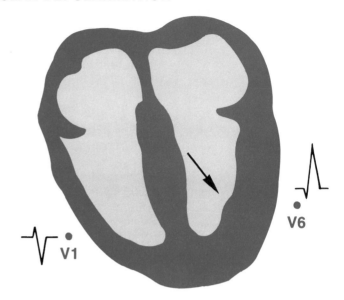

Normal Heart

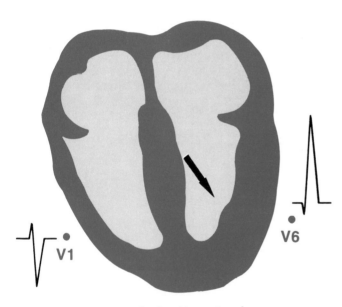

The left ventricular wall increases in thickness, increasing the positive voltages in the leads over the hypertrophied area and increasing the negative voltages in the leads opposite the hypertrophied area.

A large R wave is recorded in V_6 as the mean wave of depolarization moves toward the electrode, and a large S wave is inscribed in V_1 as the mean wave of depolarization moves away from it.

Left Ventricular Hypertrophy

Voltage criteria are used almost exclusively for the diagnosis of left ventricular hypertrophy on an ECG. We know that we will have large negative voltages in V_1 and large positive voltages in I, aVL, V_5, and V_6. The standard for recognition of left ventricular hypertrophy is:

S wave in V_1 + R wave in V_5 ≥ 35 mm
   or
R wave in aVL ≥ 11 mm
   or
R wave in V_5 or V_6 > 27 mm

Repolarization changes, in the form of ST depression and asymmetrical T wave inversion, are often present in the left heart leads, although the reasons for these changes are not entirely clear.

REPOLARIZATION CHANGES WITH LEFT VENTRICULAR HYPERTROPHY

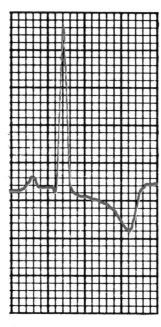

I

Left axis deviation may also be present because of the increased voltages over the left side of the heart.

LEFT VENTRICULAR HYPERTROPHY

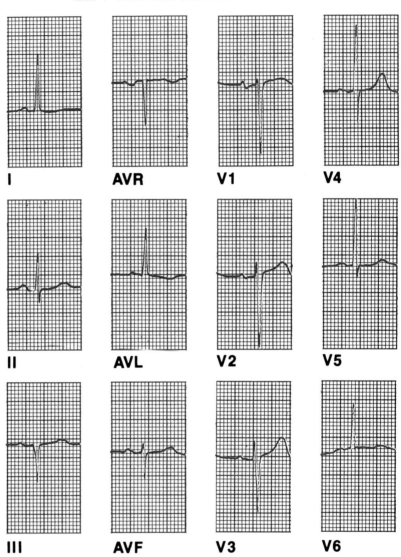

I	AVR	V1	V4
II	AVL	V2	V5
III	AVF	V3	V6

Right ventricular hypertrophy. An increase in the size of the walls of the right ventricle is called *right ventricular hypertrophy.* When the wall of the right ventricle increases in thickness, it can equal or exceed the thickness of the left ventricle. If it does not surpass the left ventricular thickness, then right ventricular hypertrophy may go unnoticed on an ECG. If the hypertrophy becomes severe, leads V_1 and V_2 will increase their R wave voltages, as the initial wave of depolarization moves toward the hypertrophied ventricle. The increase in the muscle thickness of the right ventricular wall increases the voltages in the leads over the hypertrophied area.

VENTRICULAR DEPOLARIZATION

The left ventricular wall is thicker than the right causing the mean QRS vector to point leftward, rendering a large R wave in V_6 as the mean wave of depolarization moves toward the electrode, and recording a large S wave in V_1 as the mean wave of depolarization moves away from the electrode.

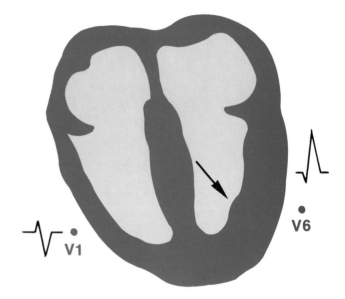

Normal Heart

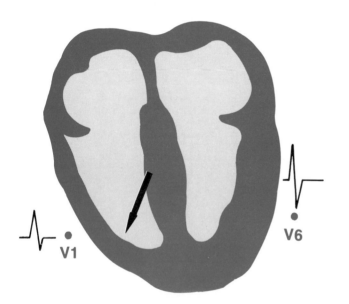

Right Ventricular Hypertrophy

The right ventricular wall increases in thickness, increasing the positive voltages in the leads over the hypertrophied area and increasing the negative voltages in the leads opposite the hypertrophied area.

A large R wave is recorded in V_1 as the mean wave of depolarization moves toward the electrode and a large S wave is inscribed in V_6 as the mean wave of depolarization moves away from it.

Voltage is one of the two criteria used for recognition of right ventricular hypertrophy:

R wave ≥ S wave in V_1
   or
R wave in V_1 + S wave in V_6 ≥ 11 mm

Repolarization changes are often present in the right heart leads in the forms of ST depression and asymmetrical T wave inversion.

REPOLARIZATION CHANGES WITH RIGHT VENTRICULAR HYPERTROPHY

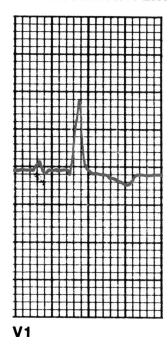

V1

The second criteria necessary for right ventricular hypertrophy is right axis deviation of +90° or greater. The axis shifts to the right in response to the greater amount of vectors present over the right ventricle.

RIGHT VENTRICULAR HYPERTROPHY

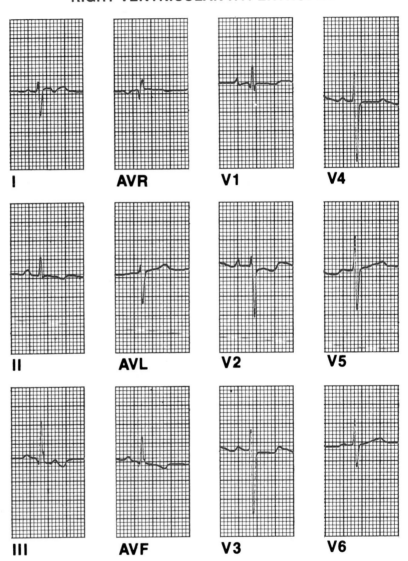

I   AVR   V1   V4

II   AVL   V2   V5

III   AVF   V3   V6

Biventricular hypertrophy. An increase in the size of both the left and right ventricular walls is called *biventricular hypertrophy.* An enlargement of both ventricles may manifest voltage criteria for left ventricular hypertrophy with a QRS axis of +90° or greater, demonstrated by large voltages in leads II, III, and AVF, although ECG recognition of this abnormality is extremely difficult because biventricular hypertrophy tends to normalize a tracing.

BIVENTRICULAR HYPERTROPHY

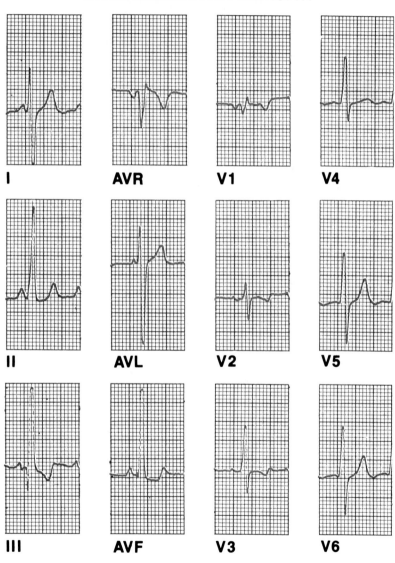

LEFT ATRIAL HYPERTROPHY

ECG Leads to Check for Left Atrial Hypertrophy

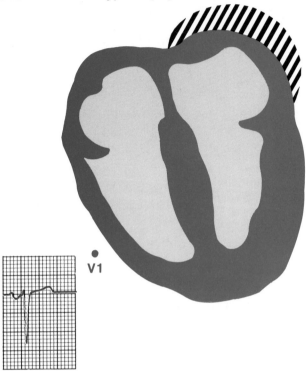

V1

Criterion

Terminal portion of P wave in $V_1 \geq -1$ mm

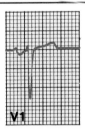

V1

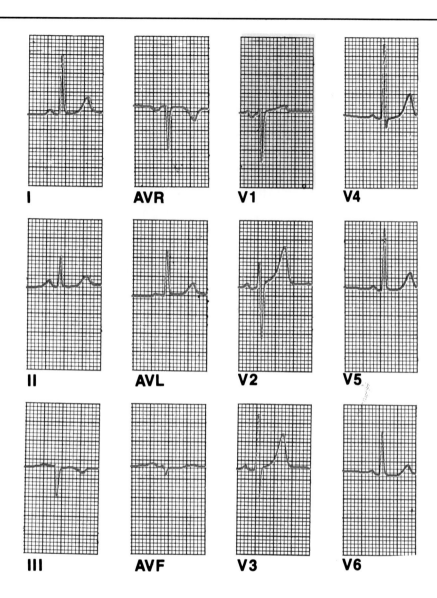

I   AVR   V1   V4

II   AVL   V2   V5

III   AVF   V3   V6

RIGHT ATRIAL HYPERTROPHY

ECG Leads to Check for Right Atrial Hypertrophy

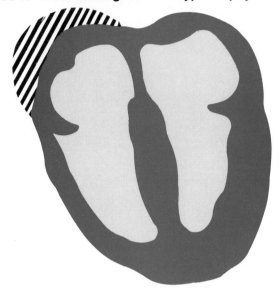

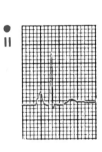

Criterion

Tall peaked P wave ≥ 2.5 mm in lead II

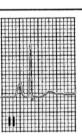

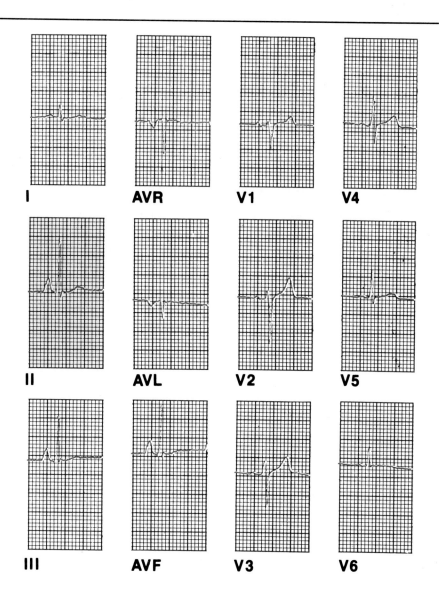

I
AVR
V1
V4

II
AVL
V2
V5

III
AVF
V3
V6

BIATRIAL HYPERTROPHY

ECG Leads to Check for Biatrial Hypertrophy

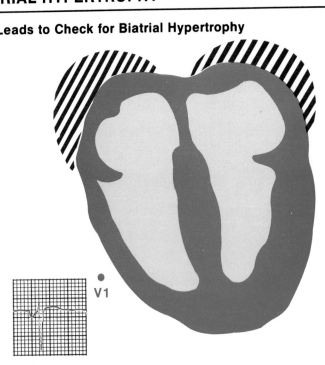

Criteria

1. Terminal portion of P wave in $V_1 \geq -1$ mm

2. Tall peaked P wave ≥ 2.5 mm in lead II

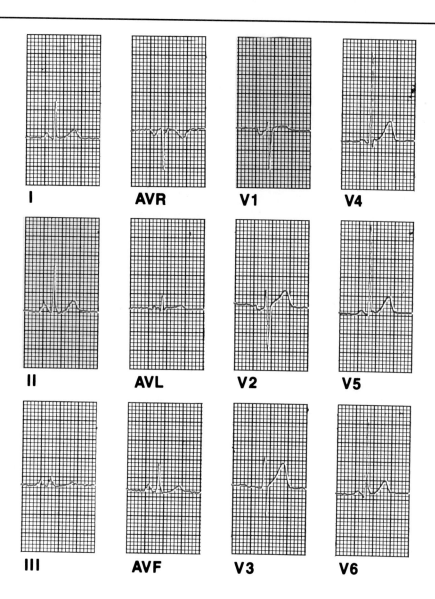

I AVR V1 V4

II AVL V2 V5

III AVF V3 V6

HYPERTROPHY

LEFT VENTRICULAR HYPERTROPHY

ECG Leads to Check for Left Ventricular Hypertrophy

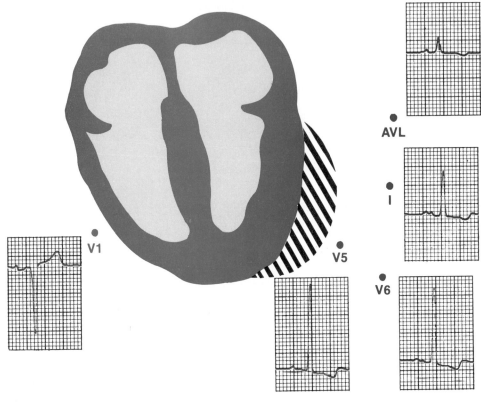

Criteria

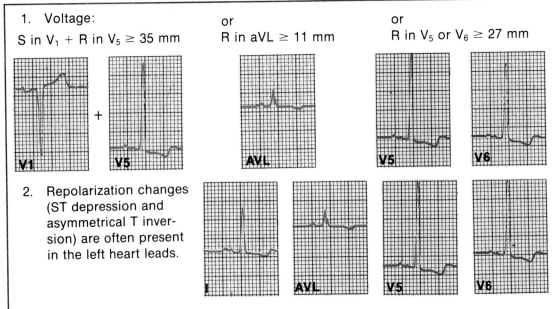

1. Voltage:
   S in V_1 + R in $V_5 \geq 35$ mm   or   R in aVL ≥ 11 mm   or   R in V_5 or $V_6 \geq 27$ mm

2. Repolarization changes (ST depression and asymmetrical T inversion) are often present in the left heart leads.

3. Left axis deviation may be present.

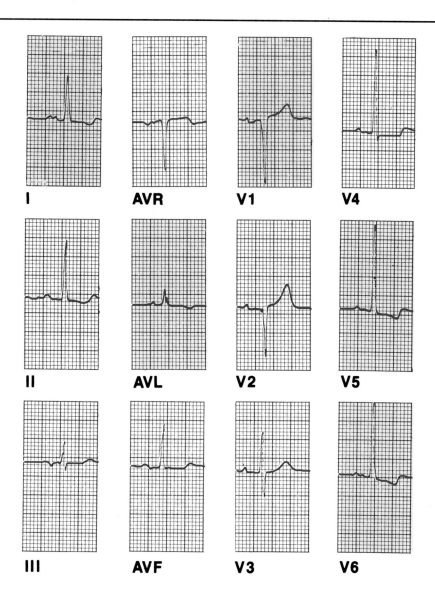

I AVR V1 V4

II AVL V2 V5

III AVF V3 V6

RIGHT VENTRICULAR HYPERTROPHY

ECG Leads to Check for Right Ventricular Hypertrophy

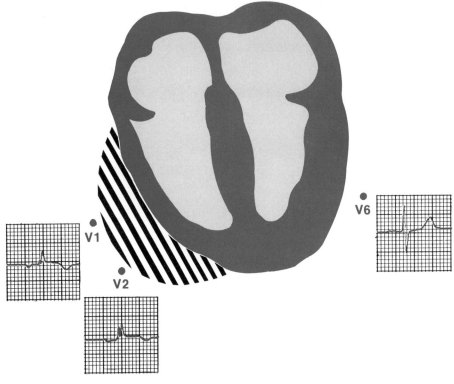

Criteria

1. Voltage:
   R wave $\geq$ S in V_1 or   R in V_1 + S in V_6 $\geq$ 11 mm

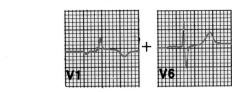

2. Right axis deviation of $+90°$ or greater

3. Repolarization changes (ST depression and asymmetrical T inversion) are often present in the right heart leads.

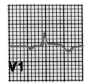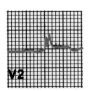

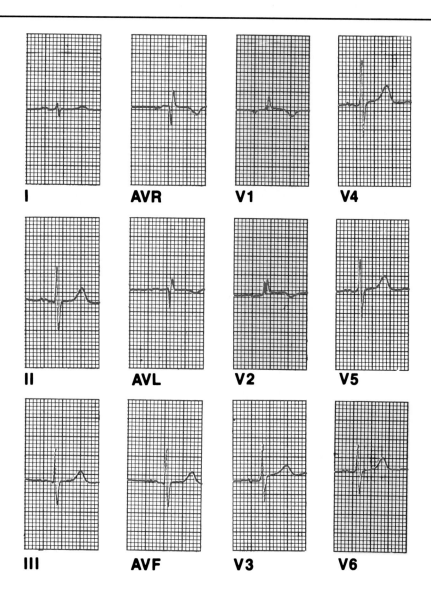

I AVR V1 V4

II AVL V2 V5

III AVF V3 V6

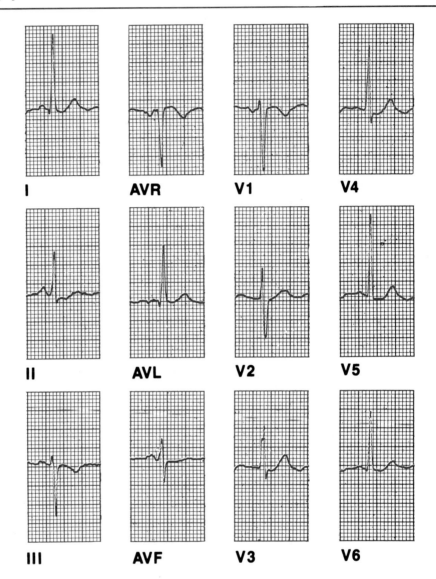

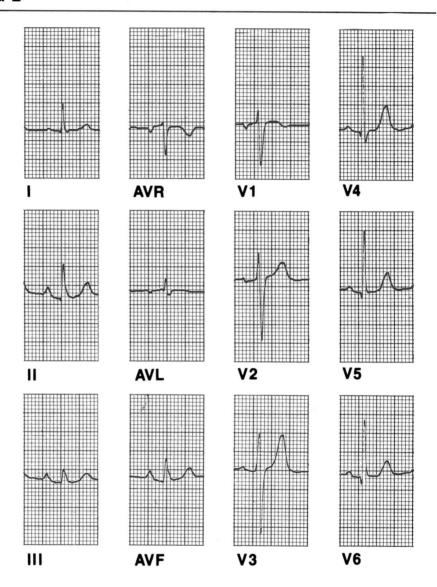

I	AVR	V1	V4
II	AVL	V2	V5
III	AVF	V3	V6

HYPERTROPHY

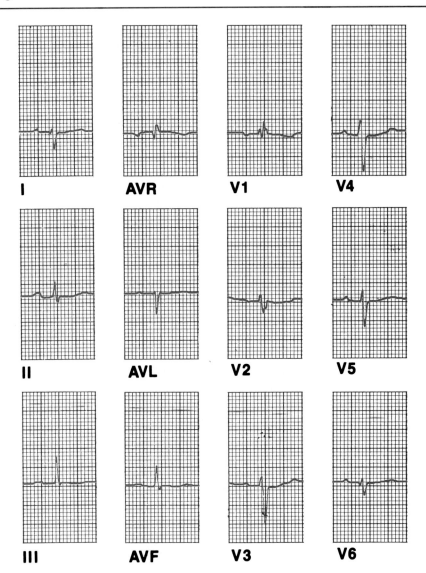

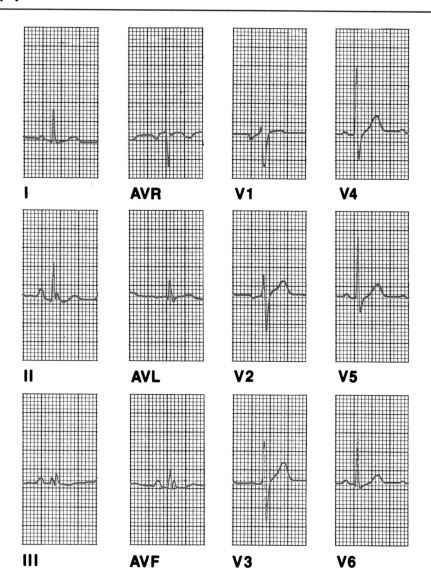

I	AVR	V1	V4
II	AVL	V2	V5
III	AVF	V3	V6

HYPERTROPHY

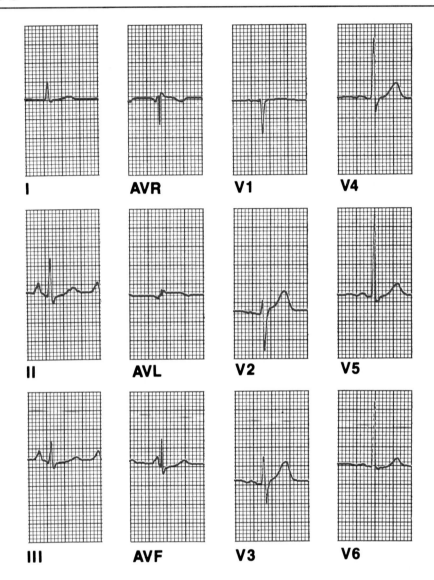

I	AVR	V1	V4
II	AVL	V2	V5
III	AVF	V3	V6

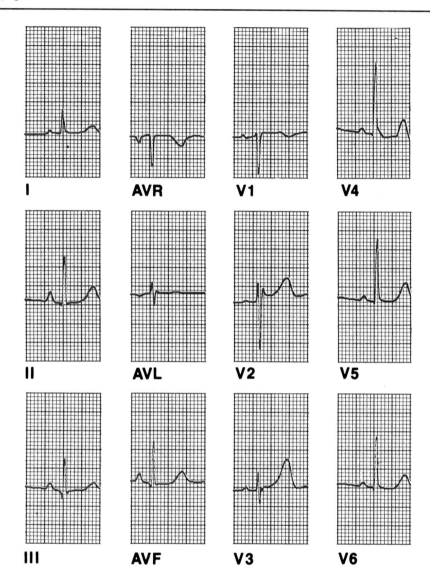

I	AVR	V1	V4
II	AVL	V2	V5
III	AVF	V3	V6

HYPERTROPHY

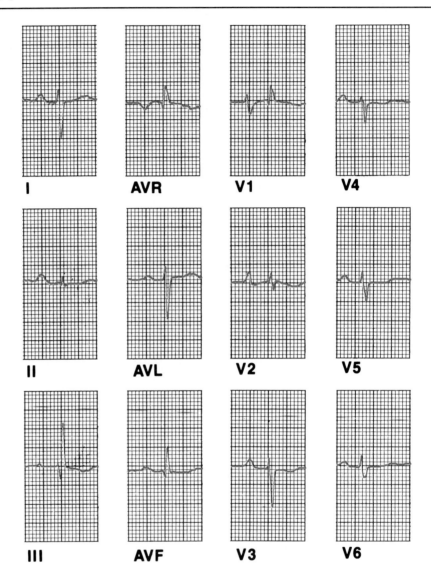

I AVR V1 V4

II AVL V2 V5

III AVF V3 V6

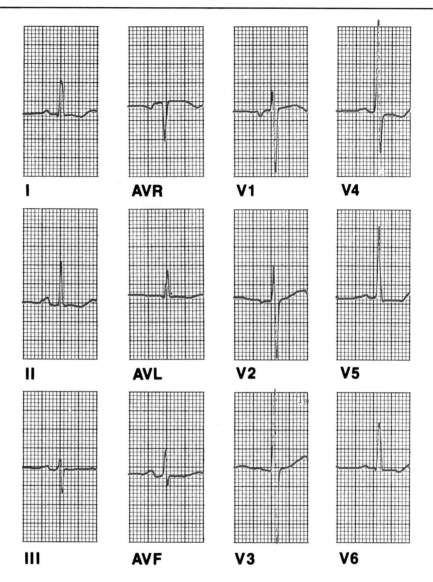

I AVR V1 V4

II AVL V2 V5

III AVF V3 V6

HYPERTROPHY

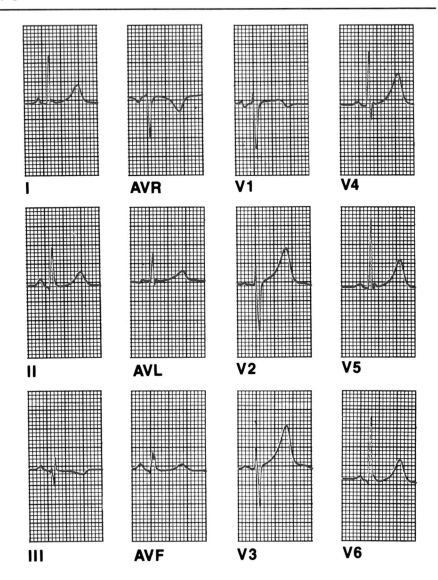

I   AVR   V1   V4

II   AVL   V2   V5

III   AVF   V3   V6

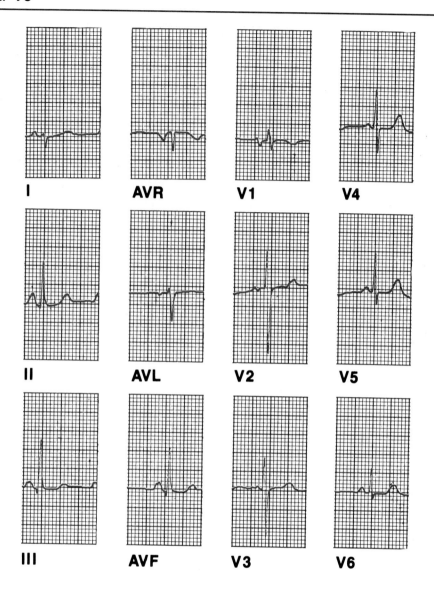

I   AVR   V1   V4

II   AVL   V2   V5

III   AVF   V3   V6

HYPERTROPHY

REVIEW ECG ANSWERS

1. Left atrial hypertrophy and left ventricular hypertrophy
2. Left atrial hypertrophy
3. First degree AV block and right ventricular hypertrophy
4. Left atrial hypertrophy
5. Right atrial hypertrophy
6. Right atrial hypertrophy
7. First degree AV block, right ventricular hypertrophy, and left atrial hypertrophy
8. Left atrial hypertrophy and left ventricular hypertrophy
9. Left atrial hypertrophy
10. Biatrial hypertrophy and right ventricular hypertrophy

Intraventricular Conduction Disturbances

An intraventricular conduction disturbance is an abnormal conduction of an electrical impulse in one or more of the conduction pathways below the bundle of His: (1) right bundle branch, (2) left bundle branch, (3) left anterior fascicle, or (4) left posterior fascicle.

BUNDLE BRANCH BLOCK

Right bundle branch block. A delay or blockage of conduction in the right bundle branch is called *right bundle branch block.* A normal cardiac impulse is initiated in the sinus node, travels through and depolarizes the atria, and transverses the AV node and bundle of His. The cardiac impulse then proceeds down the left bundle, initiates septal activation, and attempts to move down the right bundle at the same time. Upon finding the right bundle branch blocked, the electrical impulse advances through the left bundle into the anterior and posterior fascicles and into the Purkinje fibers of the left ventricle. The electrical impulse will then travel from the left ventricle across the septum, into the right ventricle, and will initiate depolarization.

The initial activation in the ventricles during right bundle branch block remains the same as that of the normal heart, since the septum depolarizes from left to right via the left bundle branch system. Lead V_1 will have an initial R wave inscribed and lead I will have a Q wave recorded. The left ventricle depolarizes first, unopposed by the right, and inscribes an S wave while the forces of depolarization are moving away from the V_1 electrode, and lead I records an R wave as the wave of depolarization moves toward it. Finally, the right ventricle depolarizes, unopposed by the left. As the wave of depolarization moves toward the V_1 electrode an R' wave is inscribed, and as the wave of depolarization moves away from lead I, an S wave is displayed.

VENTRICULAR DEPOLARIZATION

The initial activation in the ventricles is rightward and in the direction of V_1, resulting in a small R wave in V_1 as the wave of depolarization moves toward it, and a small Q in V_6 as the wave of depolarization moves away from the electrode. Left and right ventricular depolarization occur almost simultaneously, demonstrating a mean QRS vector directed leftward and inferiorly toward V_6, inscribing a large R wave, and away from V_1, displaying a deep S wave in that lead.

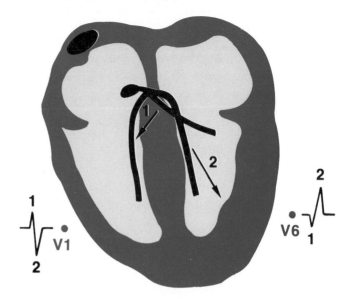

Normal Heart

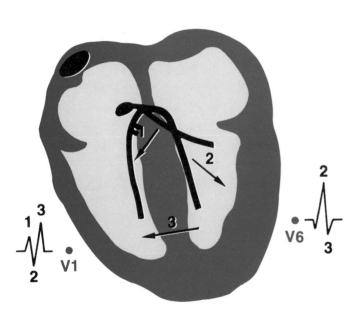

Right Bundle Branch Block

Initial ventricular depolarization is normal, resulting in a small R in V_1 and a small Q in V_6. Because of the blockage in the right bundle branch, the left ventricle depolarizes first, recording an S wave in V_1 as the wave of depolarization moves away from the electrode and an R wave in V_6 as the wave of depolarization moves toward it. The right ventricle is then depolarized abnormally across the interventricular septum, recording an R' in V_1 as the wave of depolarization again travels toward that electrode, and an S wave in V_6 as the wave of depolarization travels away from it. Because of delay in conduction in the right ventricle, the terminal portion of the QRS is widened, resulting in a QRS of .12 second or greater.

INTRAVENTRICULAR CONDUCTION DISTURBANCES

The characteristic findings of right bundle branch block are a QRS that is .12 second or greater in duration, a predominantly positive QRS in V_1, a wide S wave in lead I, and ST depression and T wave inversion, representing repolarization changes occurring with right bundle branch block. In the presence of right bundle branch block, right ventricular hypertrophy should not be diagnosed.

QRS CONFIGURATIONS

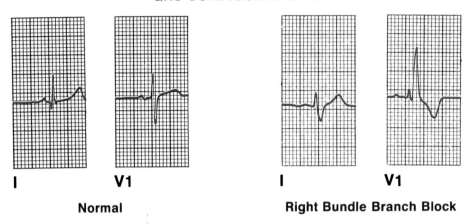

I   V1   I   V1

Normal   **Right Bundle Branch Block**

RIGHT BUNDLE BRANCH BLOCK

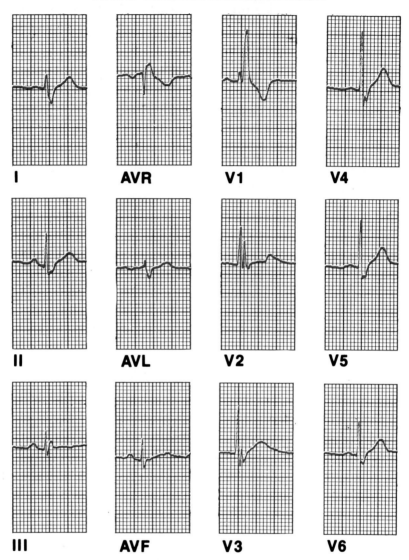

I   AVR   V1   V4

II   AVL   V2   V5

III   AVF   V3   V6

INTRAVENTRICULAR CONDUCTION DISTURBANCES

Left bundle branch block. Delay or blockage of conduction in the main left bundle branch is called *left bundle branch block.* A cardiac impulse begins in the sinus node and depolarizes the atria, travels through the AV node and the bundle of His, and arrives at the left and right bundle branches. The impulse proceeds down the right bundle branch and attempts to move down the left bundle branch. On finding the left side blocked, the wave of depolarization travels down the right bundle and initiates depolarization through the Purkinje fibers and travels across the septum to depolarize the left ventricle.

The initial activation in the ventricles during left bundle branch block is greatly changed from that of the normal heart. The septum is unable to be depolarized from left to right and is depolarized from right to left by way of the right bundle branch. Normal septal Q waves will not be seen in leads I, aVL, V_5, and V_6. Lead V_1 may show a small Q wave as the initial wave of depolarization moves away from it. The right ventricle depolarizes first, sometimes inscribing a small R wave in V_1 as the wave of depolarization moves toward it. Often, the small Q wave or R wave in V_1 will be absent, leaving only a QS wave. Lastly, the left ventricle depolarizes, unopposed by the right, and a large S wave is inscribed in V_1 as the wave of depolarization moves away from the electrode.

VENTRICULAR DEPOLARIZATION

The initial activation in the ventricles is rightward and in the direction of V_1, resulting in a small R wave in V_1 as the wave of depolarization moves toward it, and a small Q in V_6 as the wave of depolarization moves away from the electrode. Left and right ventricular depolarization occur almost simultaneously, demonstrating a mean QRS vector directed leftward and inferiorly toward V_6, inscribing a large R wave, and away from V_1, displaying a deep S wave in that lead.

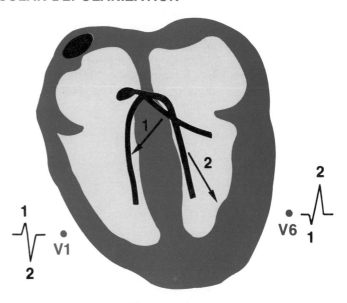

Normal Heart

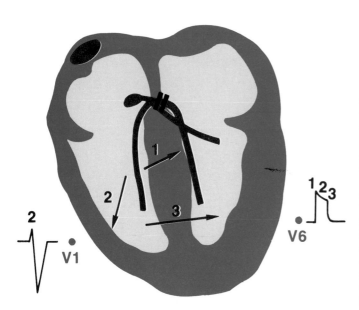

Left Bundle Branch Block

Because the left bundle branch is blocked, the septum depolarizes in a rightward direction, traveling toward V_6 and recording an R wave in it, and away from V_1, inscribing a tiny Q wave, which is often not visible. The right ventricle depolarizes first, inscribing a small R wave in V_1 as the wave of depolarization moves toward the electrode, and an S wave or slurred R wave in V_6 as the wave of depolarization moves away from it. The left ventricle is then depolarized abnormally through the interventricular septum, recording a deep S wave in V_1 as the wave of depolarization moves away from the electrode, and an R' in V_6 as the wave of depolarization moves toward it. Because of delay in conduction through the left ventricle, the entire QRS complex is widened to .12 second or greater.

INTRAVENTRICULAR CONDUCTION DISTURBANCES

The characteristic hallmarks of left bundle branch block are a widened and bizarre QRS complex that is .12 second or greater in duration, and a QRS that is predominantly negative in V_1. Septal Q waves will be absent in leads I, aVL, V_5, and V_6. ST depression and T wave inversion, representing repolarization changes of left bundle branch block, will be seen. Left ventricular hypertrophy should not be diagnosed in the presence of left bundle branch block.

V_1 QRS CONFIGURATIONS

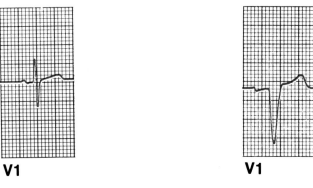

V1

Normal

V1

Left Bundle Branch Block

LEFT BUNDLE BRANCH BLOCK

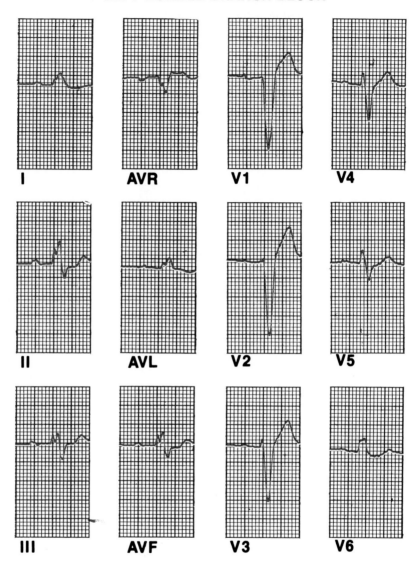

HEMIBLOCK

Left anterior hemiblock. Delay or blockage of the anterior fascicle of the left bundle branch is called *left anterior hemiblock*. The electrical impulse arrives at the bundle of His after depolarizing the atria and traveling through the AV node. The impulse then travels to the right and left bundle branches and is blocked at the anterior division of the left bundle. The depolarization wave travels down the posterior fascicle and through the connection of Purkinje fibers between the two fascicles, the anterior portion of the left ventricle is depolarized.

The initial activation in the ventricles remains the same as in a normal heart, since the septum depolarizes from left to right via the remaining fascicle. Lead I will have a Q wave recorded as the wave of depolarization moves away from the electrode, and lead III will display an initial R wave as the wave of depolarization moves toward it. The right bundle branch depolarizes normally, and the left bundle branch depolarizes in a slightly different way. The posterior fascicle depolarizes the posterior portion of the left ventricle, and then the anterior portion is depolarized with a minimum of delay through the connections of the Purkinje fibers with the posterior division. The main wave of depolarization will be orientated superiorly toward lead I rather than leftward and laterally. This will produce an R wave in lead I and an S wave in lead III.

VENTRICULAR DEPOLARIZATION

The initial activation in the ventricles is rightward and in the direction of III, resulting in a small R in III as the wave of depolarization moves toward it, and a small Q wave in I as the wave of depolarization travels away from the electrode. Left and right ventricular depolarization occur almost simultaneously, demonstrating a mean QRS vector directed leftward toward lead I, inscribing an R wave, and inferiorly toward lead III also displaying an R wave, or variable patterns of R and S waves.

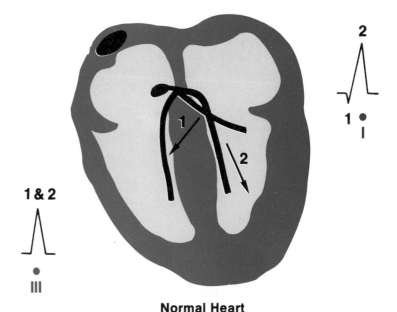

Normal Heart

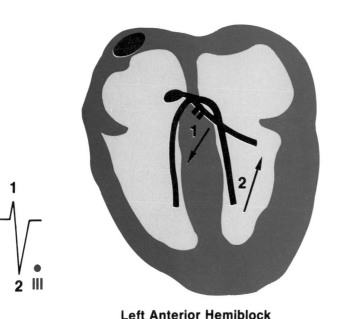

Left Anterior Hemiblock

The initial activation in the ventricles is usually rightward, traveling toward III and inscribing a small R wave, and away from I, recording a small Q wave. The mean QRS vector remains leftward but because of the blockage in the left anterior branch, the mean QRS vector now becomes superior, resulting in a deep S wave in III as the wave of depolarization moves away from the electrode, and an R wave in I as the wave of depolarization travels toward it.

INTRAVENTRICULAR CONDUCTION DISTURBANCES

The characteristic signs of left anterior hemiblock are an axis shift to −40° or greater, a small Q wave in Lead I and no evidence of inferior infarction (see Chapter 12). If left anterior hemiblock is present the voltage criteria for left ventricular hypertrophy in aVL is increased to 16 mm or greater.

LEFT ANTERIOR HEMIBLOCK

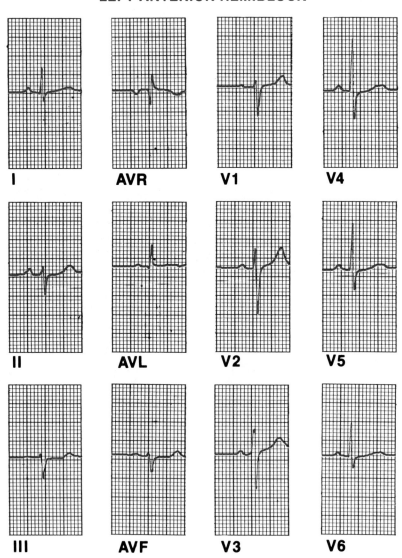

I AVR V1 V4

II AVL V2 V5

III AVF V3 V6

Left posterior hemiblock. Delay or blockage of the posterior fascicle of the left bundle branch is called *left posterior hemiblock*. The electrical impulse arrives at the right and left bundle branches after traveling through normal conduction pathways. Conduction proceeds down the right bundle branch normally. Conduction is either delayed or blocked at the posterior division of the left bundle branch, so the impulse travels down the anterior fascicle and through the connection of Purkinje fibers between the two fascicles; the posterior portion of the left ventricle is depolarized.

Although septal activation still occurs, the majority of the forces of initial depolarization in the ventricles are moving superiorly and leftward by way of the anterior fascicle toward lead I, recording an R wave; and are moving away from lead III, displaying a Q wave.

After the superior portion of the left ventricle is depolarized by way of the anterior fascicle, the inferior portion will be depolarized by the connections of purkinje fibers between the two fascicles. The main wave of depolarization is projected inferiorly, toward lead III, recording an R wave; and away from lead I, producing an S wave.

VENTRICULAR DEPOLARIZATION

The initial activation in the ventricles is rightward and in the direction of III, resulting in a small R in III as the wave of depolarization moves toward it, and a small Q wave in I as the wave of depolarization travels away from the electrode. Left and right ventricular depolarization occur almost simultaneously, demonstrating a mean QRS vector directed leftward toward lead I, inscribing an R wave, and inferiorly toward lead III also displaying an R wave, or variable patterns of R and S waves.

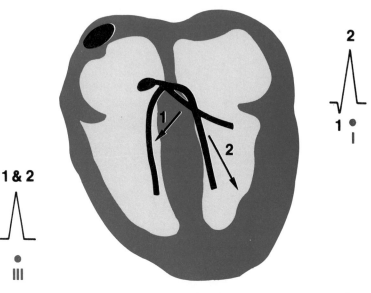

Normal Heart

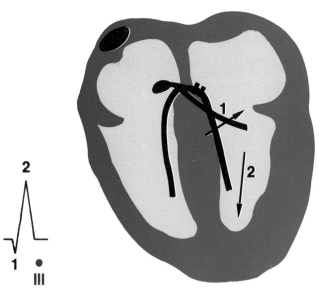

Left Posterior Hemiblock

The initial activation in the ventricles is leftward, traveling toward I and recording a small R wave, and away from III, inscribing a Q wave. The mean QRS vector becomes rightward, and because of the blockage in the left posterior branch, the mean QRS vector now becomes inferior, resulting in a large R wave in III as the wave of depolarization moves toward it, and a deep S wave in I as the wave of depolarization travels away from the electrode.

The criteria for recognition of left posterior hemiblock are an axis shift to +120° or greater, a small Q wave in Lead III and no evidence of right ventricular hypertrophy.

LEFT POSTERIOR HEMIBLOCK

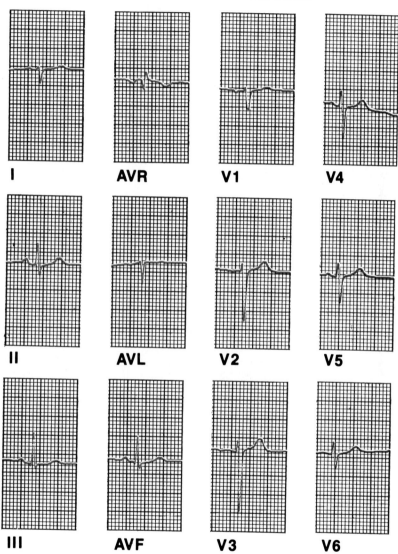

INTRAVENTRICULAR CONDUCTION DISTURBANCES

145

BIFASCICULAR BLOCK

Bifascicular block indicates blockage in more than one conducting fascicle in the ventricles:

1. Right bundle branch block and left anterior hemiblock
2. Right bundle branch block and left posterior hemiblock
3. Right or left bundle branch block with prolonged AV conduction in the remaining fascicle (first degree AV block—PR .20 second or greater)
4. Alternating right and left bundle branch block

1. Right bundle branch block and left anterior hemiblock are characterized by a QRS .12 second or greater, a wide S wave and a small Q wave in Lead I and a predominantly positive QRS in V_1, and a QRS axis of $-40°$ or greater.

RIGHT BUNDLE BRANCH BLOCK AND LEFT ANTERIOR HEMIBLOCK

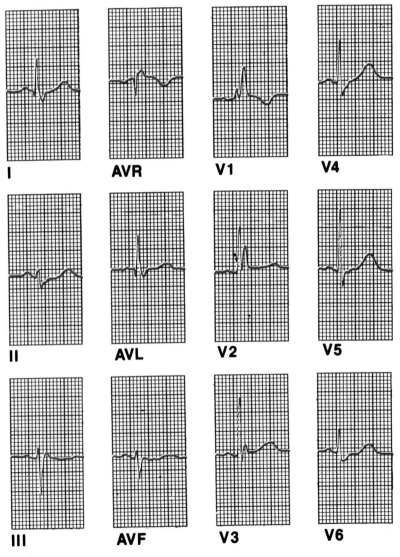

I	AVR	V1	V4
II	AVL	V2	V5
III	AVF	V3	V6

2. Right bundle branch block and left posterior hemiblock are recognized by a QRS .12 second or greater, a wide S wave in lead I and a predominantly positive QRS in V_1, a QRS axis $+120°$ or greater, and a small Q wave in Lead III.

RIGHT BUNDLE BRANCH BLOCK AND LEFT POSTERIOR HEMIBLOCK

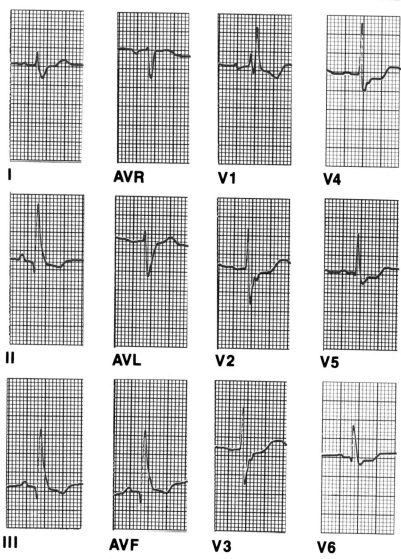

I	AVR	V1	V4
II	AVL	V2	V5
III	AVF	V3	V6

INTRAVENTRICULAR CONDUCTION DISTURBANCES

3. Right or left bundle branch block with first degree AV block is seen as right bundle branch block with a QRS .12 second or greater, a wide S wave in lead I and a predominantly positive QRS in V_1 with a PR .20 second or greater; or it may be seen as left bundle branch block with a QRS .12 second or greater, a predominantly negative QRS in V_1, no evidence of septal Q waves in leads I, aVL, V_5 and V_6, and a PR .20 second or greater. If the first degree AV block represents delay in conduction in the AV node rather than in the remaining conducting fascicle, bifascicular block would not be present.

RIGHT BUNDLE BRANCH BLOCK AND FIRST DEGREE AV BLOCK

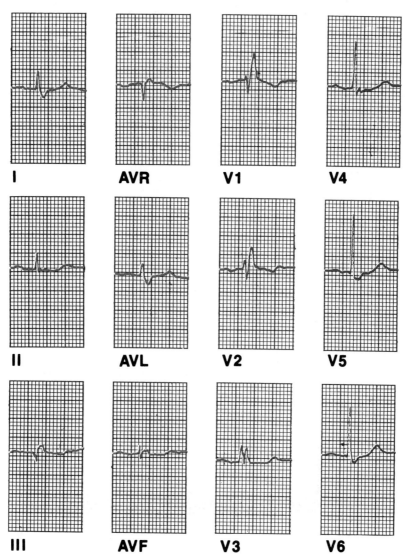

LEFT BUNDLE BRANCH BLOCK AND FIRST DEGREE AV BLOCK

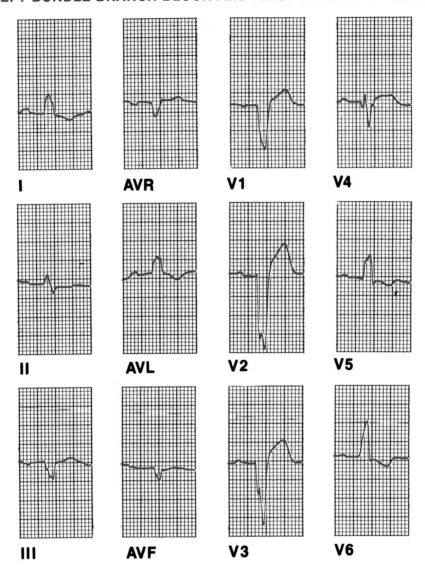

I AVR V1 V4

II AVL V2 V5

III AVF V3 V6

4. Alternating left and right bundle branch block is characterized by a left bundle branch block configuration, varying with a right bundle branch block pattern.

NONSPECIFIC INTRAVENTRICULAR CONDUCTION DISTURBANCE

A conduction abnormality located in the ventricles that is characterized by a QRS .12 second or greater that does not conform to either the left or right bundle branch block pattern is called *nonspecific intraventricular conduction disturbance.*

NONSPECIFIC INTRAVENTRICULAR CONDUCTION DELAY

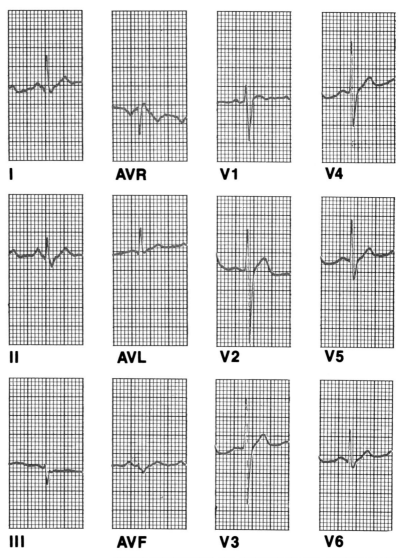

INTRAVENTRICULAR CONDUCTION DISTURBANCES

RIGHT BUNDLE BRANCH BLOCK

ECG Leads to Check for Right Bundle Branch Block

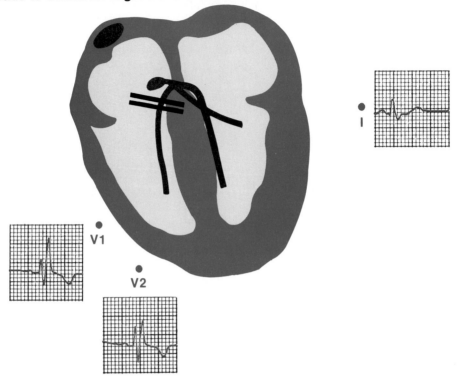

Criteria

1. QRS interval
   .12 second or greater

2. QRS predominantly
   positive in V_1

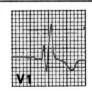

3. Wide S
   in lead I

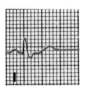

4. Repolarization
   changes

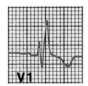

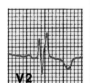

5. Do not diagnose right ventricular hypertrophy in the presence of right bundle branch block.

HOW TO QUICKLY AND ACCURATELY MASTER ECG INTERPRETATION

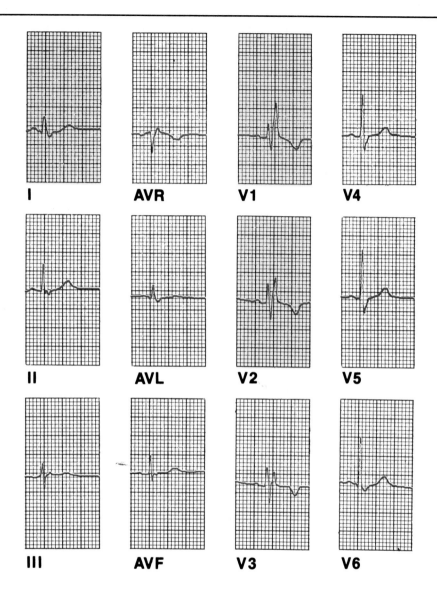

I AVR V1 V4

II AVL V2 V5

III AVF V3 V6

LEFT BUNDLE BRANCH BLOCK

ECG Leads to Check for Left Bundle Branch Block

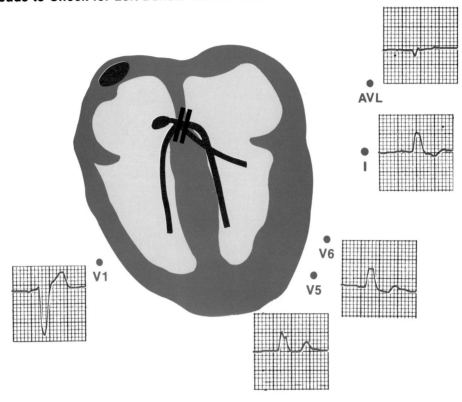

Criteria

1. QRS interval .12 second or greater

2. QRS predominantly negative in V₁

3. Absence of septal Q waves in I, avL, V₅, and V₆

4. Repolarization changes

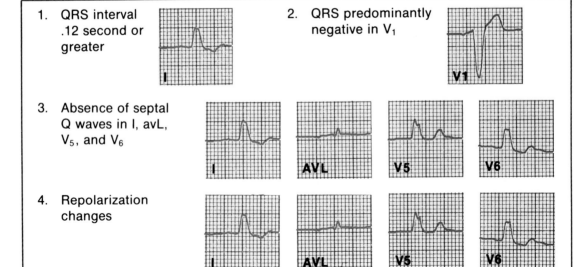

5. Do not diagnose left ventricular hypertrophy in the presence of left bundle branch block

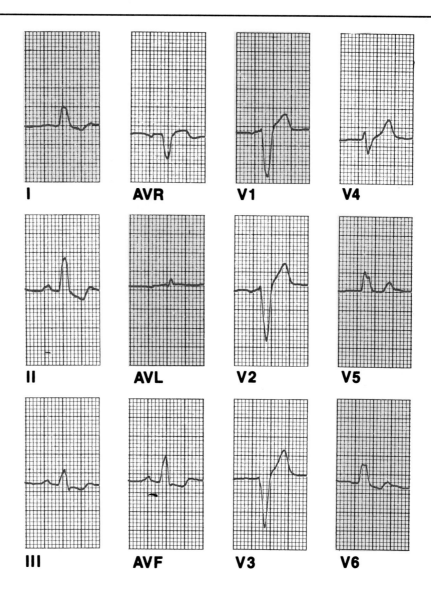

I AVR V1 V4

II AVL V2 V5

III AVF V3 V6

INTRAVENTRICULAR CONDUCTION DISTURBANCES

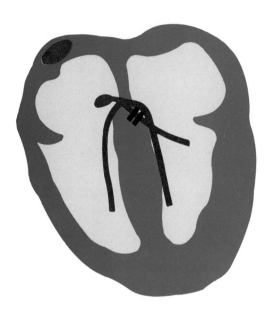

Criteria

1. Axis −40° or greater
2. No evidence of inferior infarction
3. Small Q wave in Lead I

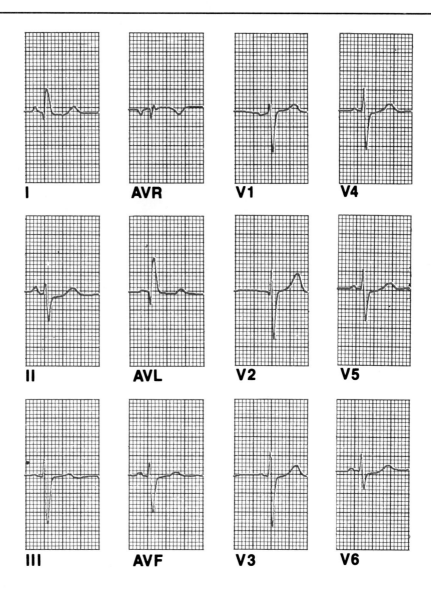

I AVR V1 V4

II AVL V2 V5

III AVF V3 V6

INTRAVENTRICULAR CONDUCTION DISTURBANCES

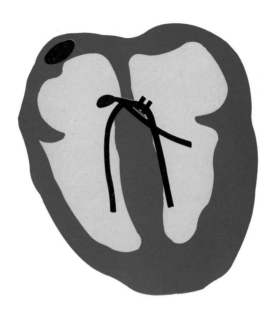

Criteria

1. Axis +120° or greater

2. No evidence of right ventricular hypertrophy

3. Small Q wave in Lead III

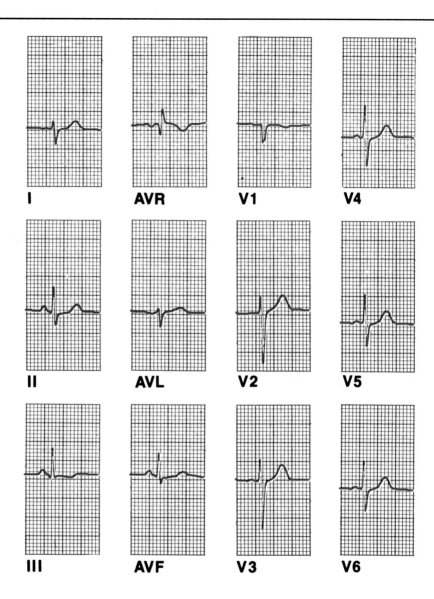

| I | AVR | V1 | V4 |

| II | AVL | V2 | V5 |

| III | AVF | V3 | V6 |

INTRAVENTRICULAR CONDUCTION DISTURBANCES

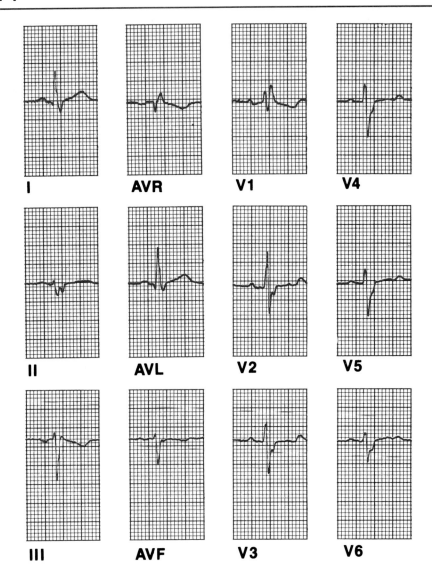

I	AVR	V1	V4
II	AVL	V2	V5
III	AVF	V3	V6

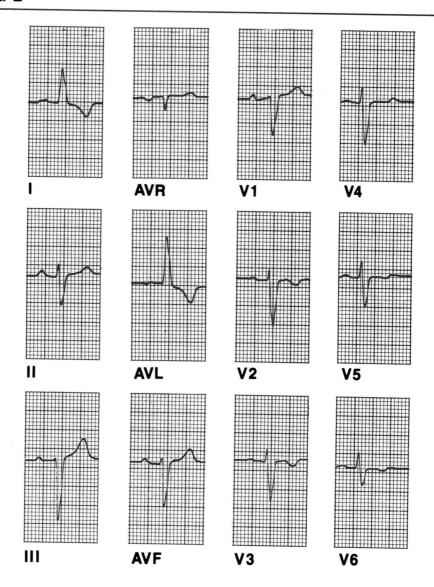

I   AVR   V1   V4

II   AVL   V2   V5

III   AVF   V3   V6

INTRAVENTRICULAR CONDUCTION DISTURBANCES

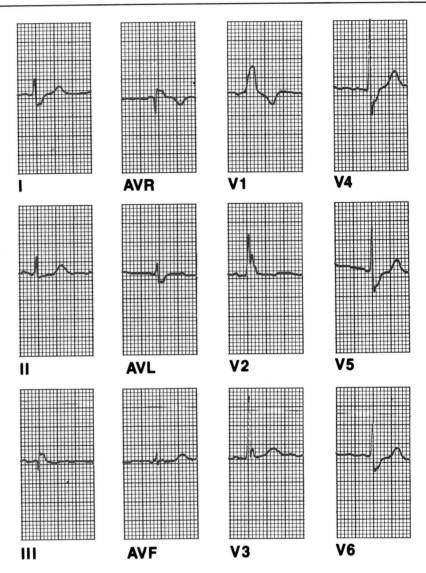

I AVR V1 V4

II AVL V2 V5

III AVF V3 V6

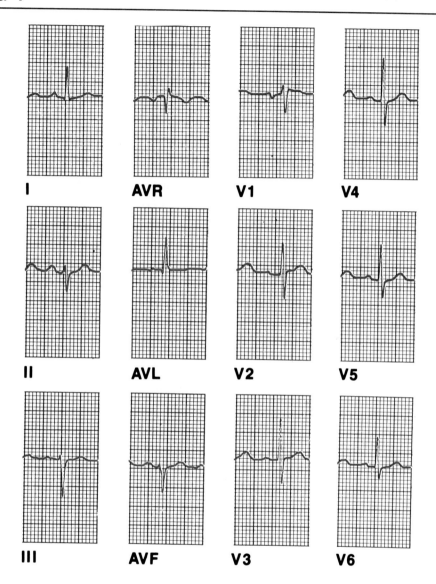

I   AVR   V1   V4

II   AVL   V2   V5

III   AVF   V3   V6

INTRAVENTRICULAR CONDUCTION DISTURBANCES

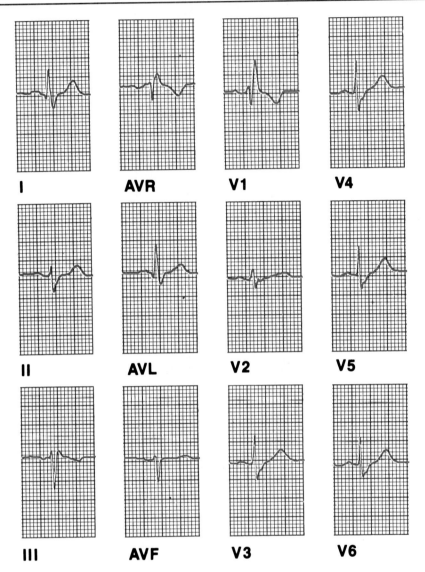

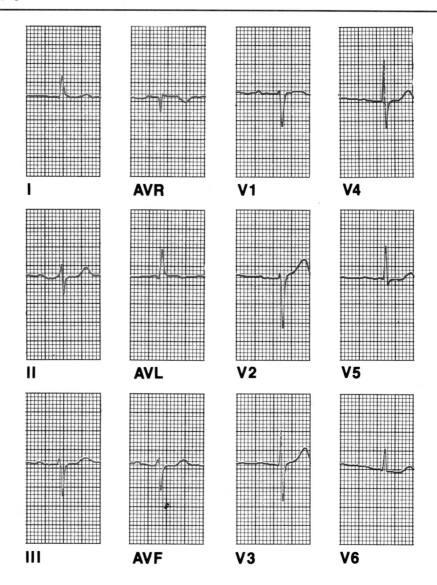

I AVR V1 V4

II AVL V2 V5

III AVF V3 V6

INTRAVENTRICULAR CONDUCTION DISTURBANCES

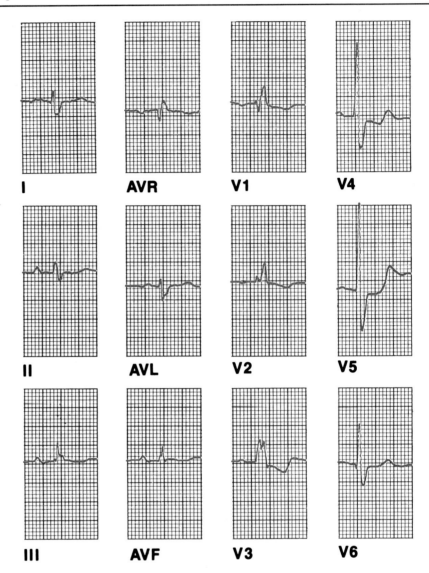

I AVR V1 V4

II AVL V2 V5

III AVF V3 V6

HOW TO QUICKLY AND ACCURATELY MASTER ECG INTERPRETATION

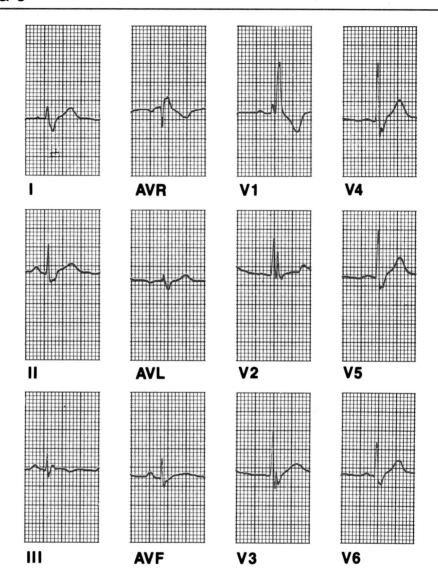

INTRAVENTRICULAR CONDUCTION DISTURBANCES

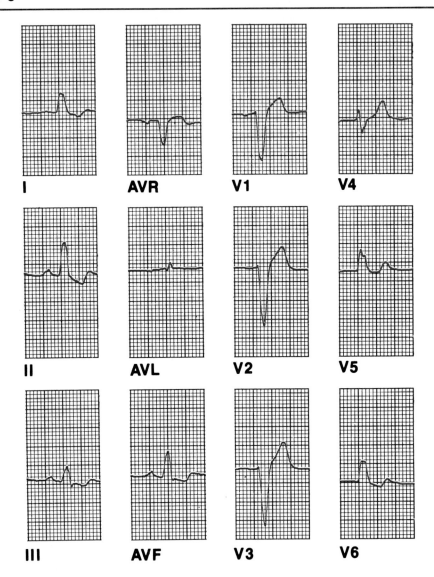

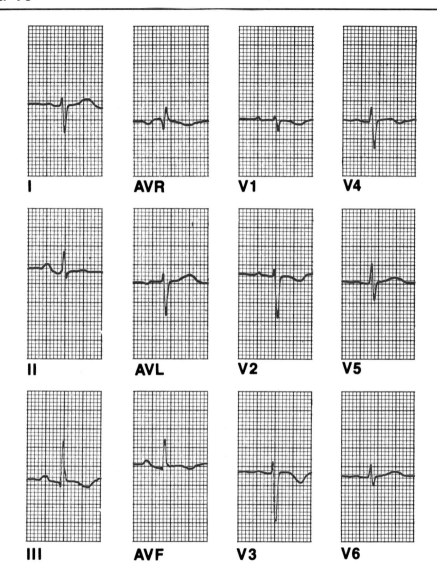

I AVR V1 V4

II AVL V2 V5

III AVF V3 V6

INTRAVENTRICULAR CONDUCTION DISTURBANCES

REVIEW ECG ANSWERS

1. Left anterior hemiblock and right bundle branch block
2. First degree AV block and left bundle branch block
3. Right bundle branch block
4. Left atrial hypertrophy and left anterior hemiblock
5. Left anterior hemiblock and right bundle branch block
6. First degree AV block and left anterior hemiblock
7. Left posterior hemiblock and right bundle branch block
8. Right bundle branch block
9. Left bundle branch block
10. First degree AV block and left posterior hemiblock

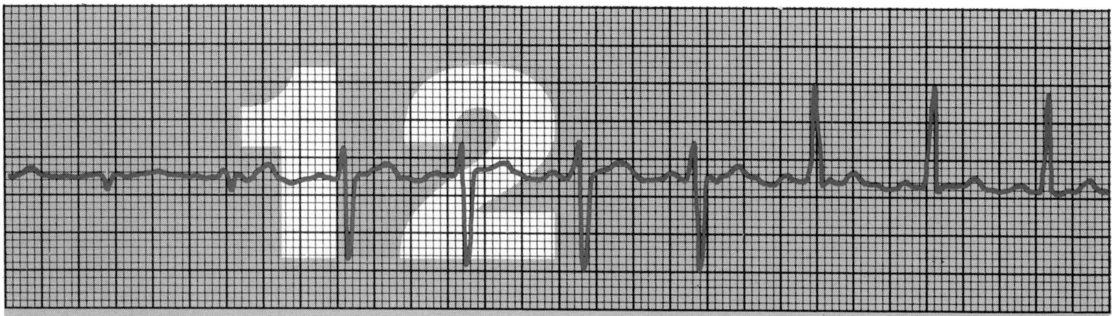

12

Ischemia, Injury, and Infarction

The heart muscle must receive a sufficient blood supply via its own network of arteries, called *coronary arteries.* The two arteries that supply the heart muscle with oxygenated blood are the left and right coronary arteries. The left coronary artery has two major branches—the circumflex branch, which travels to the upper lateral wall of the left ventricle and the left atrium, and the anterior descending branch, which courses down the anterior portion of the heart. The right coronary artery curves around the right ventricle and separates into a variable number of branches.

Variations in the branching pattern of the coronary arteries are common. Left or right coronary artery dominance denotes which artery provides the greatest portion of oxygenated blood to the base of the left ventricle. Sometimes both the left and right coronary arteries have a fairly balanced pattern of distribution of blood and neither one is considered dominant.

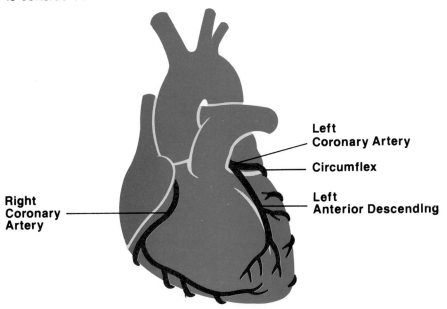

A narrowing of the coronary arteries, often caused by atherosclerosis, results in a diminished blood supply to the heart. During rest, these narrowed coronary arteries may deliver a sufficient blood supply to the heart, but with exertion the rapidly pumping thick left ventricle requires a greater blood supply, and will be the chamber to suffer by reduction in blood flow. Lack of adequate oxygenated blood results in ischemia. If the heart is without a blood supply, injury to the left heart muscle will occur. And finally, if the blood supply is not returned, death of a portion of the left ventricular muscle will occur and is termed *infarction.*

ISCHEMIA

Ischemia is a lack of sufficient oxygenated blood to the left ventricle, and is manifested on the ECG by symmetrically inverted T waves or ST depression.

ISCHEMIA

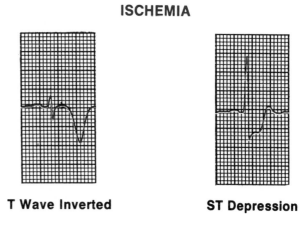

T Wave Inverted   **ST Depression**

All the ECG leads should be routinely checked for T wave inversion and ST depression. Remember, T waves are always inverted in aVR and can normally be inverted in lead III and V_1.

NORMAL ECG

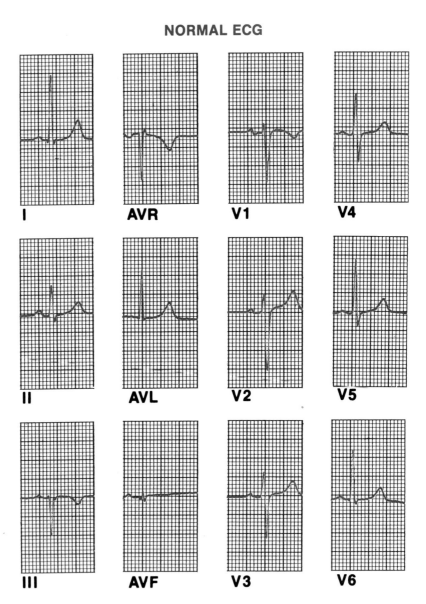

I **AVR** **V1** **V4**

II **AVL** **V2** **V5**

III **AVF** **V3** **V6**

T waves in Lead III and V_1 may be inverted.

INJURY

Injury is a stage beyond ischemia and is manifested on the ECG by ST elevation. Like ischemia, injury is a reversible process and no permanent damage necessarily occurs. All the leads on an ECG should be routinely checked for ST elevation.

ST SEGMENT ELEVATION

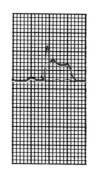

INFARCTION

Infarction is necrosis or death of tissue in a portion of the left ventricular myocardial wall, and follows the stages of ischemia and injury if an adequate blood supply is not returned. Infarction is demonstrated on an ECG by significant Q waves. In order for Q waves to be considered significant, they must either be .04 second wide or one third the height of the R wave. If neither of these conditions are met, the Q waves are not diagnostic of infarction. Septal Q waves—those normally found in lead I, aVL, V_5, and V_6—represent depolarization of the ventricular septum and are not pathologic.

Q WAVES

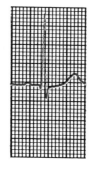

Septal Q Wave

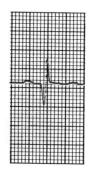

Significant Q Wave

The production of the Q wave of infarction is explained by the use of vectors. The three vectors representing ventricular depolarization in the normal heart are each averages of the electrical forces occurring in the right and left ventricles at a given time. Vector 1 represents septal and early right ventricular activation and is an average of the combined right and left ventricular forces. Vector 2 represents apical activation and is an average of combined electrical forces of the right and left ventricles. Vector 3 denotes left ventricular activation.

VENTRICULAR DEPOLARIZATION

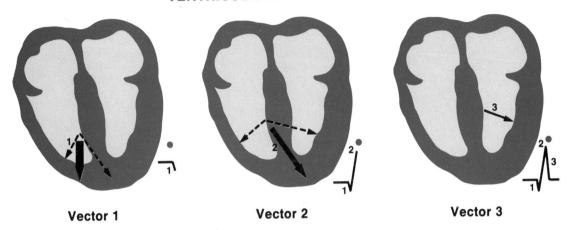

Vector 1   Vector 2   Vector 3

The three vectors representing ventricular depolarization in the normal heart are each averages of the forces occurring in the ventricles at a given time, producing a mean QRS vector moving toward the electrode, and recording a predominantly positive QRS.

With infarction, the electrical forces from the damaged left ventricle are nonexistent, so the electrical forces from the right ventricle are unopposed and a deep and wide Q wave is produced as the electrical forces move away from the electrode during activation of the infarcted area.

ORIGIN OF THE Q WAVE IN INFARCTION

VENTRICULAR DEPOLARIZATION

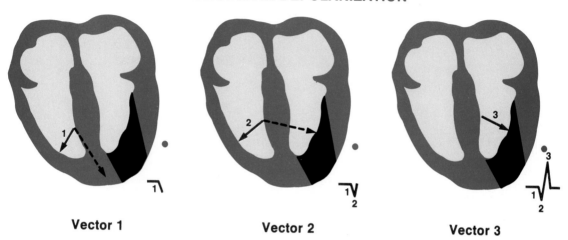

Vector 1   Vector 2   Vector 3

With infarction there are no vectors from the electrically dead area in the left ventricle. The right ventricular vectors are now unopposed and the majority of electrical activity is now traveling away from the electrode, recording a significant Q wave.

ISCHEMIA, INJURY, AND INFARCTION

When we discuss ischemia, injury, or infarction we are referring to conditions present in the left ventricle. We can be more specific and determine approximately what area of the left ventricle is being affected. The left ventricle is divided into four main locations: anterior, lateral, inferior, and posterior. Leads V_1, V_2, V_3, and V_4 are located over the anterior portion of the left ventricle. Leads I, aVL, V_5, and V_6 are placed over the lateral portion, and leads II, III, and aVF are positioned over the inferior portion of the left ventricle. No leads are placed directly over the posterior aspect of the left ventricle, but by observing the opposite or anterior wall, some determinations can be made.

INFARCT LOCATIONS IN THE LEFT VENTRICLE AND ELECTRODE POSITIONS

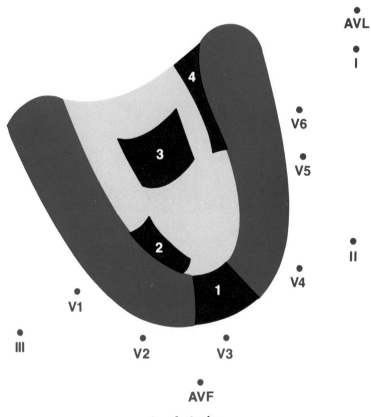

1. Anterior
2. Inferior
3. Posterior
4. Lateral

We can classify the infarcted left ventricular muscle electrically into three regions: (1) the region of infarction where the heart muscle is electrically dead and does not conduct any impulses, (2) the region of injury that immediately surrounds the infarcted area and has cell membranes which are never completely polarized, and (3) the region of ischemia in which repolarization is impaired.

INFARCTION, INJURY, AND ISCHEMIA OF THE LEFT VENTRICLE

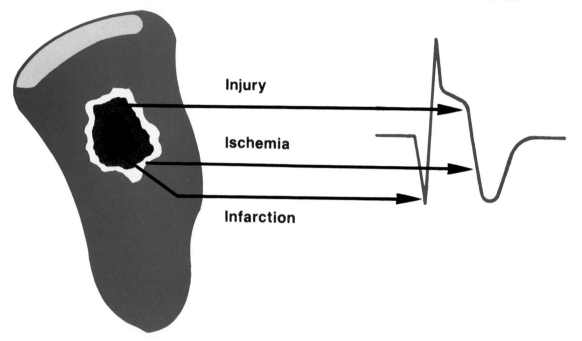

The sequence of stages in the development and evolution of a myocardial infarction usually proceeds as follows:

1. An area of left ventricular muscle is injured and ST elevation occurs in the ECG leads over the injured area.

ST ELEVATION

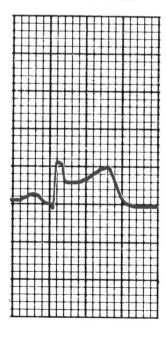

2. Q waves develop in the ECG
   leads over the infarcted area.

Q WAVE

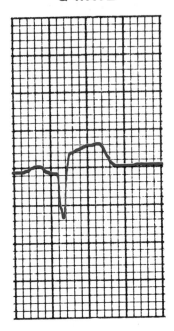

3. T wave inversion occurs in the
   ECG leads over the infarcted
   area.

**T INVERSION AND
ST ELEVATION REMAINS**

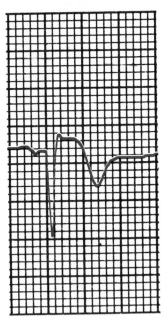

HOW TO QUICKLY AND ACCURATELY MASTER ECG INTERPRETATION

4. ST elevation returns to baseline and T waves remain inverted over the injured
myocardium.

ONLY T INVERSION REMAINS

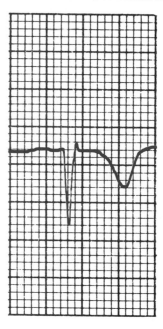

Reciprocal changes in infarction on an ECG are demonstrated by ST
depression in the leads opposite the infarcted area.

RECIPROCAL CHANGES OF INFARCTION

INFERIOR INFARCTION

ST DEPRESSION IN LEADS OPPOSITE INFARCTION

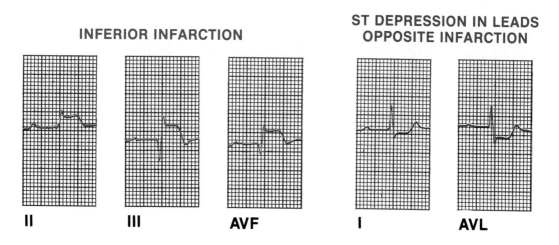

| II | III | AVF | I | AVL |

ISCHEMIA, INJURY, AND INFARCTION

We can make a determination about the age of an infarction by examining the ST segment and T waves in the leads over the infarcted area. If the ST segments are elevated, the infarction is probably acute. If the ST segments are at baseline and the T waves are inverted, we might conclude that an infarction is present with an age indeterminate. On the other hand, if the ST segments are at baseline and the T waves are upright, we might conclude that the infarction is old. It is often difficult to make exact determinations of infarction age from isolated ECGs.

ACUTE INFARCTION   **INFARCTION, AGE INDETERMINATE**   **OLD INFARCTION**

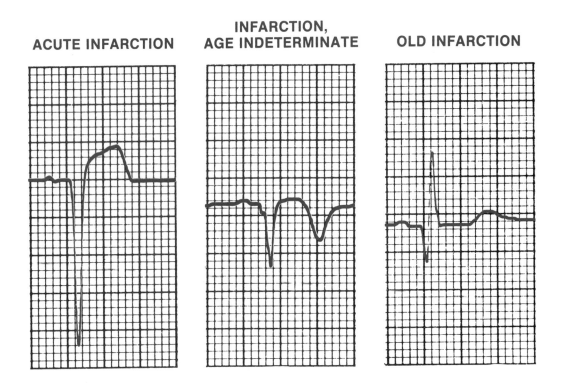

Infarction can be determined by identifying significant Q waves in at least two ECG leads for each infarct location, or by noting loss of R wave potential.

Anterlor infarction. Q waves in V_1, V_2, V_3, or V_4

ANTERIOR INFARCTION

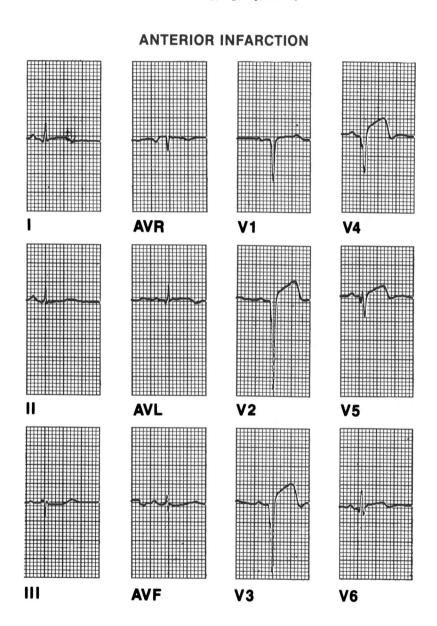

I	AVR	V1	V4
II	AVL	V2	V5
III	AVF	V3	V6

ISCHEMIA, INJURY, AND INFARCTION

Anterior septal infarction. Q waves in V_1 and V_2 only or poor R wave progression in V_1 and V_2

ANTERIOR SEPTAL INFARCTION

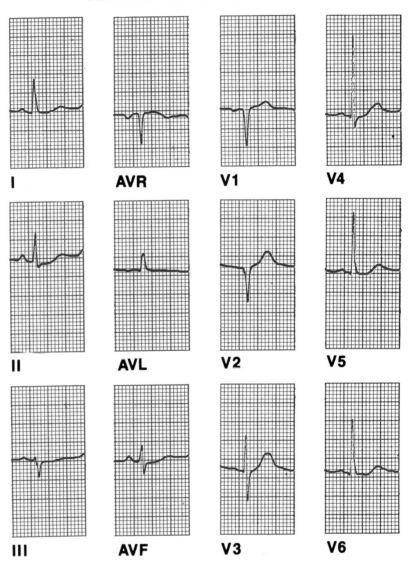

I   AVR   V1   V4

II   AVL   V2   V5

III   AVF   V3   V6

ANTERIOR SEPTAL INFARCTION

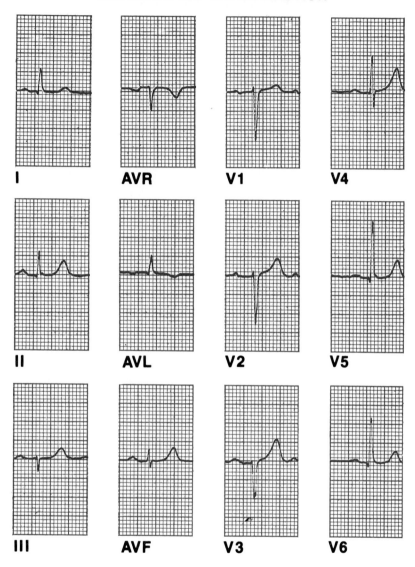

Q waves in V_1 and V_2 or poor R wave progression may also be caused by left ventricular hypertrophy. Always consider left ventricular hypertrophy to be the source of these abnormalities, but do not rule out the possibility of an anterior septal myocardial infarction.

ISCHEMIA, INJURY, AND INFARCTION

Lateral infarction. Q waves in I, aVL, V_5, or V_6

LATERAL INFARCTION

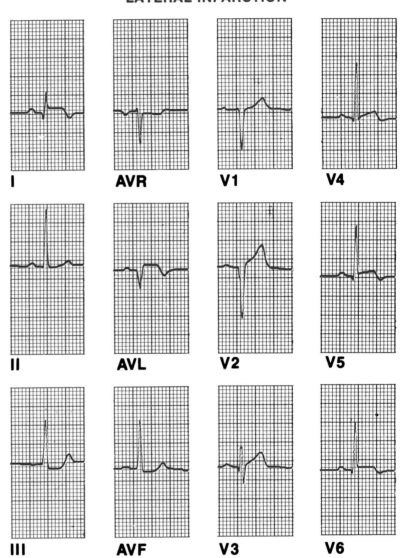

Inferior infarction. Q waves in II, III, or aVF

INFERIOR INFARCTION

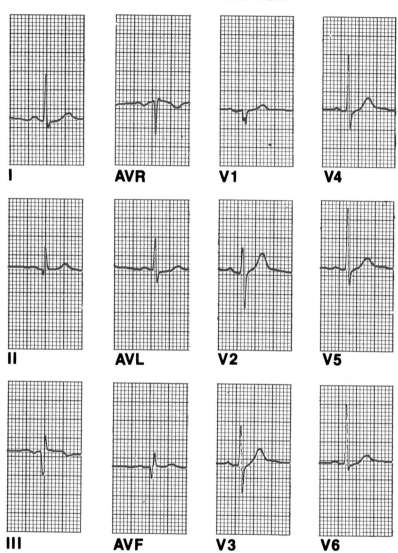

I AVR V1 V4

II AVL V2 V5

III AVF V3 V6

Posterior infarction. Tall R waves in V_1 and V_2, often accompanied by tall T waves. A posterior infarction is recognized by using the ECG leads on the opposite or anterior wall. Instead of inspecting for significant Q waves, you would inspect for the opposite effect or tall R waves. An acute posterior infarction would have depressed rather than elevated ST segments. It is difficult to determine with accuracy whether a posterior infarction is present or whether the tall R waves are a normal variant. Always suspect a posterior infarction when tall R waves are present in V_1 and V_2, accompanied by an inferior infarction.

POSTERIOR INFARCTION

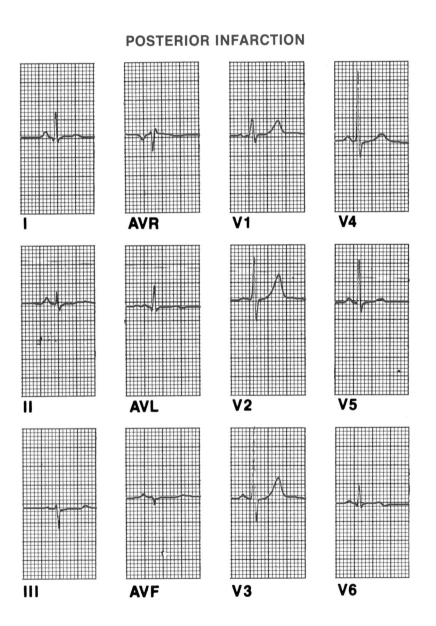

INFERIOR POSTERIOR INFARCTION

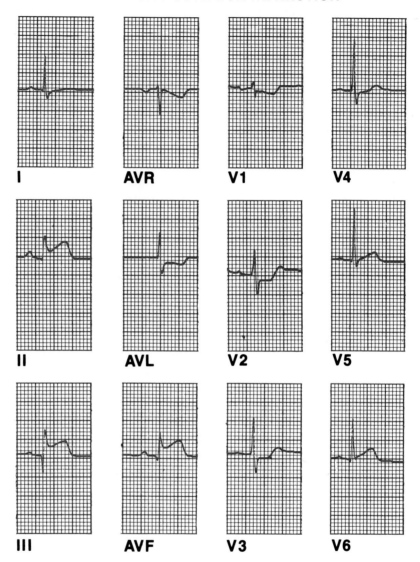

I AVR V1 V4

II AVL V2 V5

III AVF V3 V6

Infactions can occur either as isolated events or in various combinations.

ANTERIOR LATERAL INFARCTION

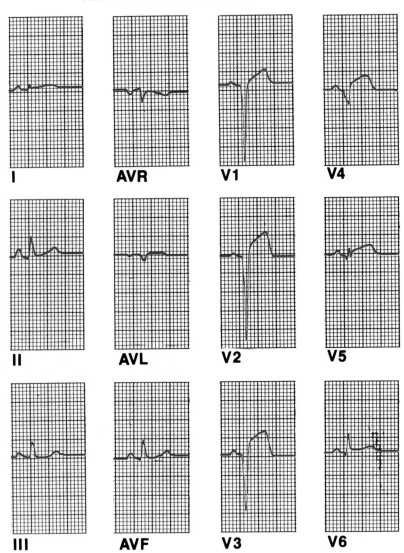

I   AVR   V1   V4

II   AVL   V2   V5

III   AVF   V3   V6

ANTERIOR, LATERAL, AND INFERIOR INFARCTION

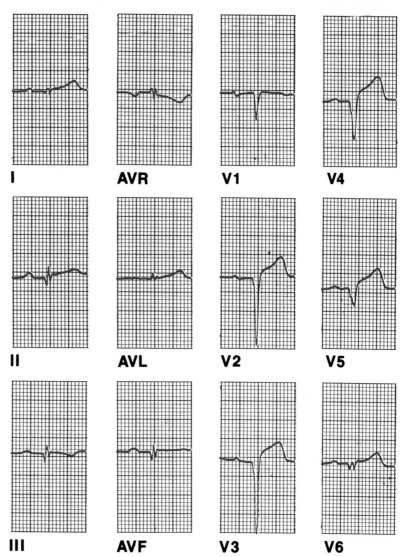

INFERIOR, POSTERIOR, AND LATERAL INFARCTION

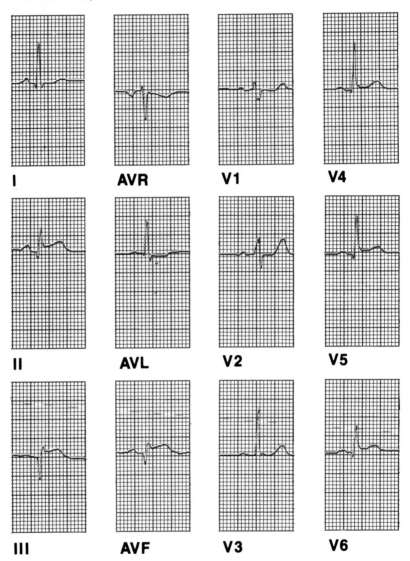

I	AVR	V1	V4
II	AVL	V2	V5
III	AVF	V3	V6

Myocardial infarction should not be diagnosed in the presence of left bundle branch block. The right ventricle depolarizes before the left ventricle in left bundle branch block, so any Q wave signifying infarction would be buried in the QRS rather than appearing at the beginning of the complex.

DO NOT DIAGNOSE INFARCTION IN THE PRESENCE OF LEFT BUNDLE BRANCH BLOCK

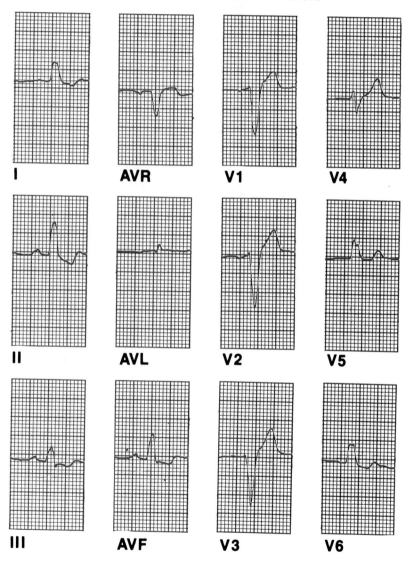

I   AVR   V1   V4

II   AVL   V2   V5

III   AVF   V3   V6

ISCHEMIA, INJURY, AND INFARCTION

ANTERIOR INFARCTION

ECG Leads to Check for Anterior Infarction

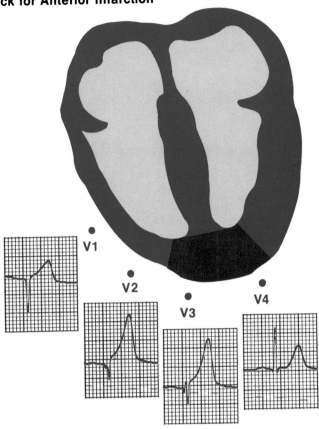

Criterion

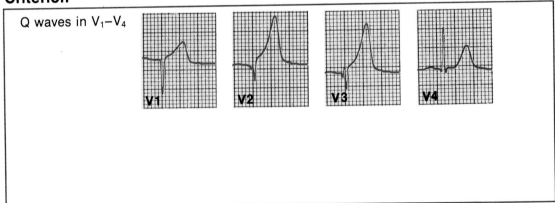

Q waves in V_1–V_4

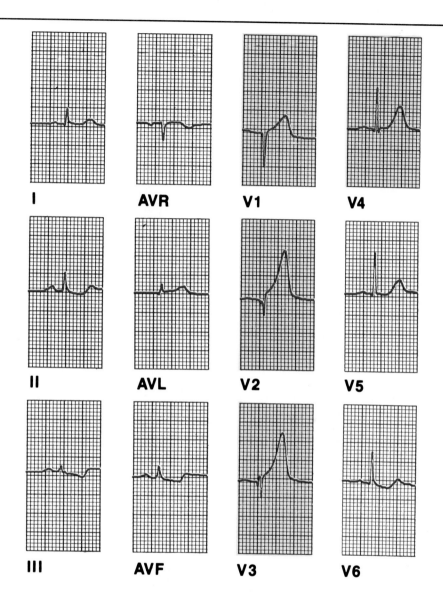

I　　　　AVR　　　　V1　　　　V4

II　　　　AVL　　　　V2　　　　V5

III　　　　AVF　　　　V3　　　　V6

ISCHEMIA, INJURY, AND INFARCTION

ANTERIOR SEPTAL INFARCTION

ECG Leads to Check for Anterior Septal Infarction

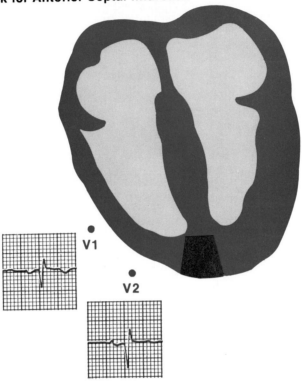

Criterion

Q waves in V_1 and V_2
   or
Poor R wave progression in V_1 and V_2

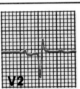

196

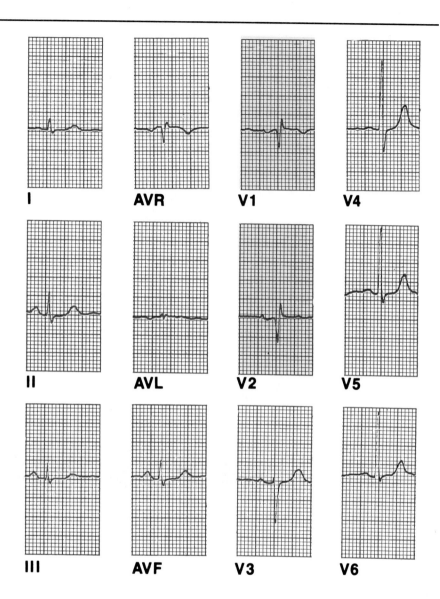

I   AVR   V1   V4

II   AVL   V2   V5

III   AVF   V3   V6

ISCHEMIA, INJURY, AND INFARCTION

LATERAL INFARCTON

ECG Leads to Check for Lateral Infarction

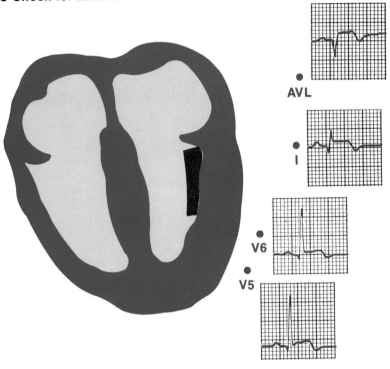

AVL

I

V6

V5

Criterion

Q waves in I, aVL, V5, and V6

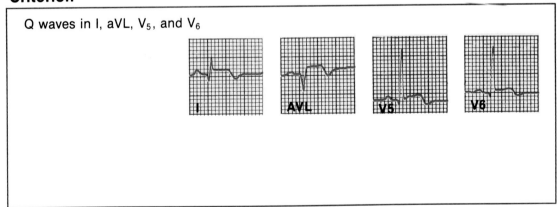

I   AVL   V5   V6

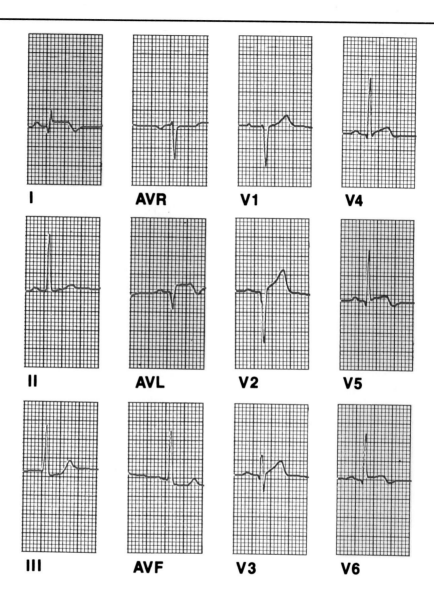

I AVR V1 V4

II AVL V2 V5

III AVF V3 V6

ISCHEMIA, INJURY, AND INFARCTION

INFERIOR INFARCTION

ECG Leads to Check for Inferior Infarction

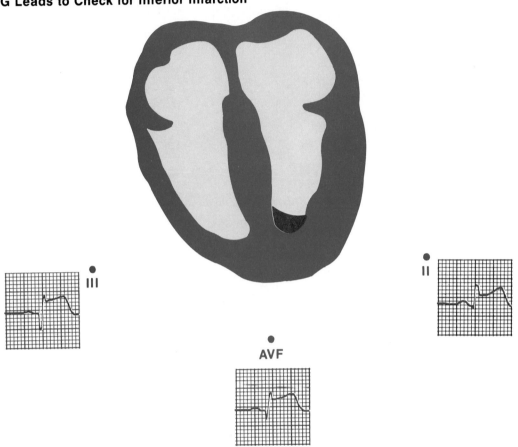

Criterion

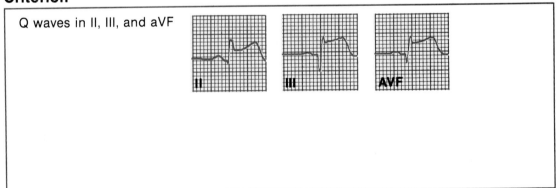

Q waves in II, III, and aVF

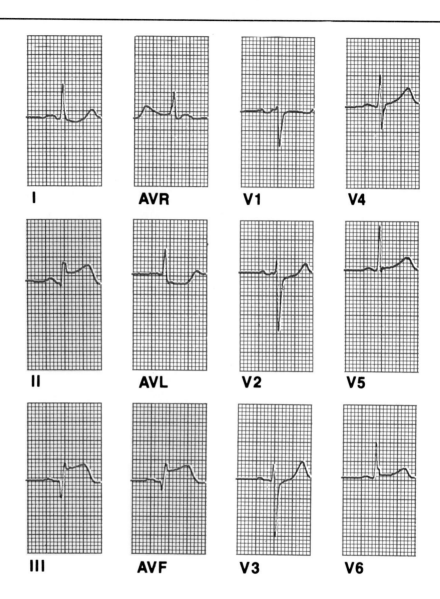

I AVR V1 V4

II AVL V2 V5

III AVF V3 V6

ISCHEMIA, INJURY, AND INFARCTION

POSTERIOR INFARCTION

ECG Leads to Check for Posterior Infarction

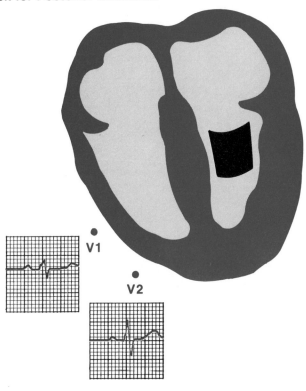

Criterion

Tall R waves in V_1 and V_2 often accompanied by tall T waves

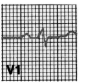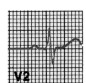

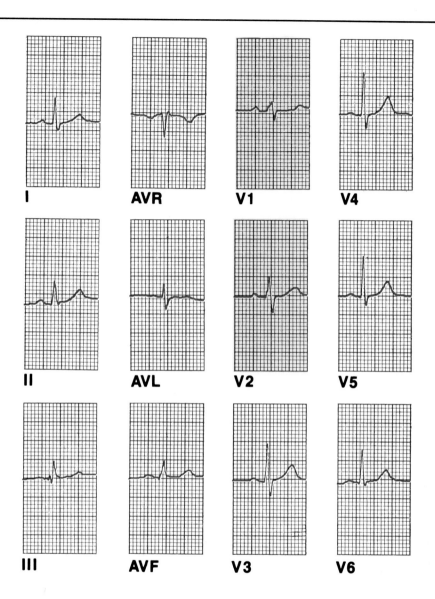

I AVR V1 V4

II AVL V2 V5

III AVF V3 V6

ISCHEMIA, INJURY, AND INFARCTION

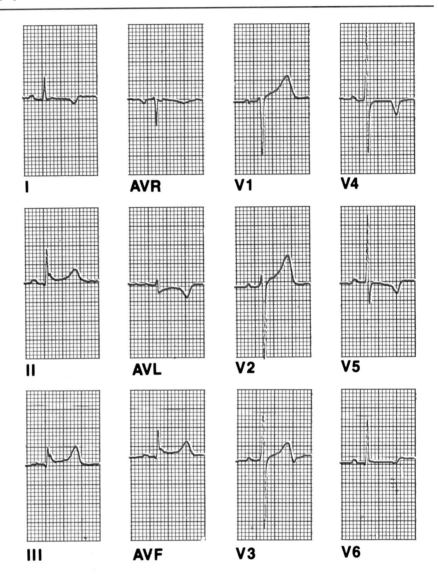

I AVR V1 V4

II AVL V2 V5

III AVF V3 V6

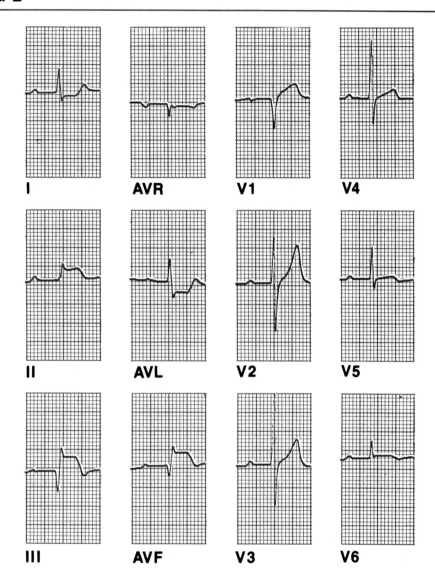

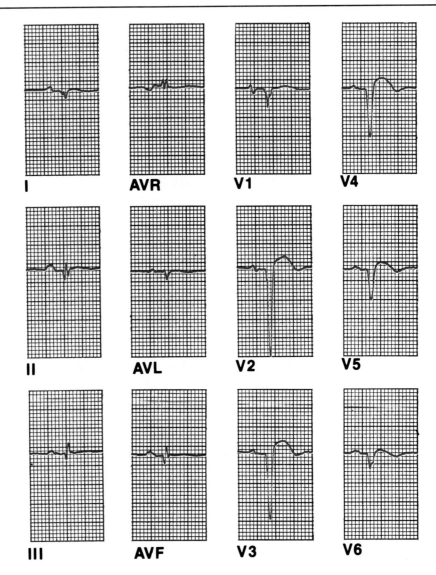

I	AVR	V1	V4
II	AVL	V2	V5
III	AVF	V3	V6

REVIEW ECG 4

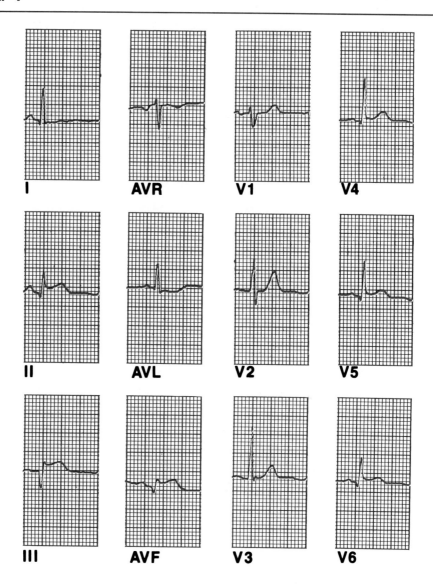

I AVR V1 V4

II AVL V2 V5

III AVF V3 V6

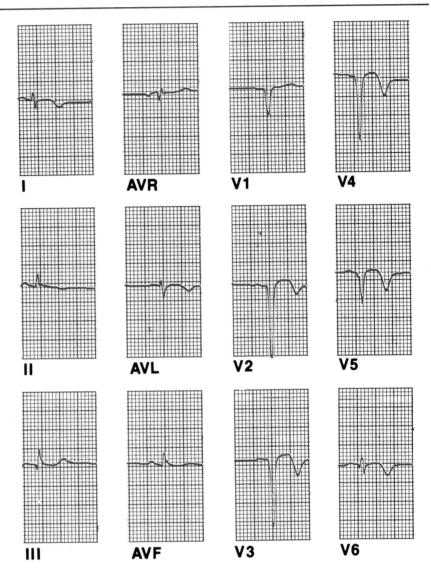

I AVR V1 V4

II AVL V2 V5

III AVF V3 V6

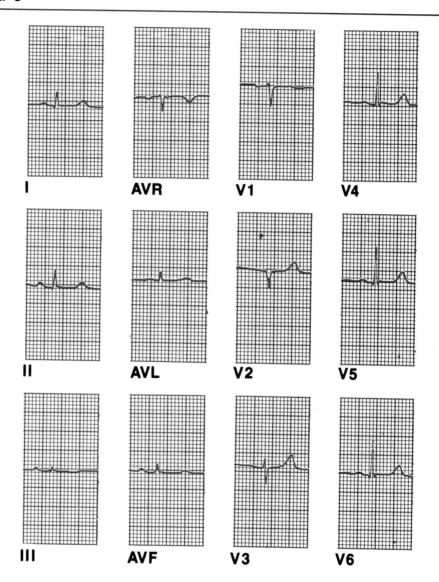

I	AVR	V1	V4
II	AVL	V2	V5
III	AVF	V3	V6

ISCHEMIA, INJURY, AND INFARCTION

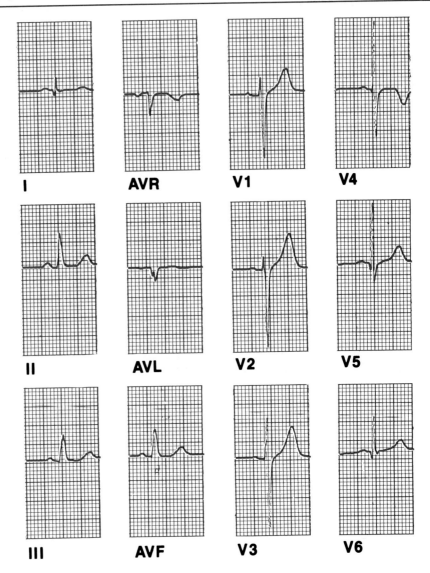

I AVR V1 V4
II AVL V2 V5
III AVF V3 V6

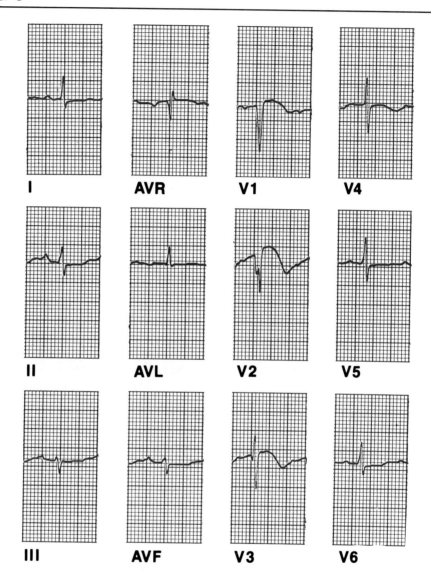

I   AVR   V1   V4

II   AVL   V2   V5

III   AVF   V3   V6

ISCHEMIA, INJURY, AND INFARCTION

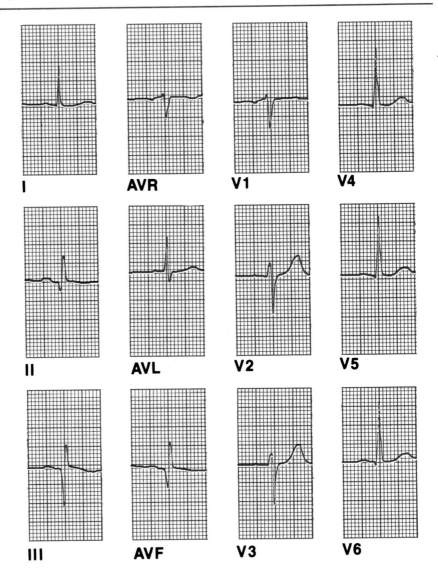

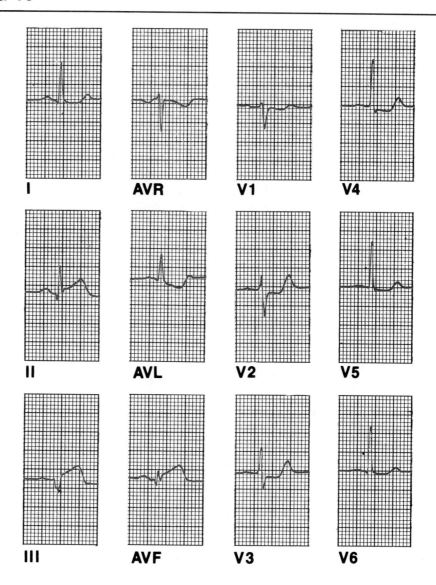

I AVR V1 V4

II AVL V2 V5

III AVF V3 V6

ISCHEMIA, INJURY, AND INFARCTION

REVIEW ECG ANSWERS

1. Anterolateral ischemia, inferior injury
2. First degree AV block, acute inferior infarction with reciprocal ST depression
3. Left atrial hypertrophy, acute anterolateral infarction, old inferior infarction
4. Acute inferior infarction, consider acute posterior infarction
5. Anterolateral infarction, age indeterminate
6. Anterior septal infarction, old
7. Lateral infarction, age indeterminate
8. Anterior septal infarction, age indeterminate
9. Inferior infarction, age indeterminate
10. Acute inferior infarction

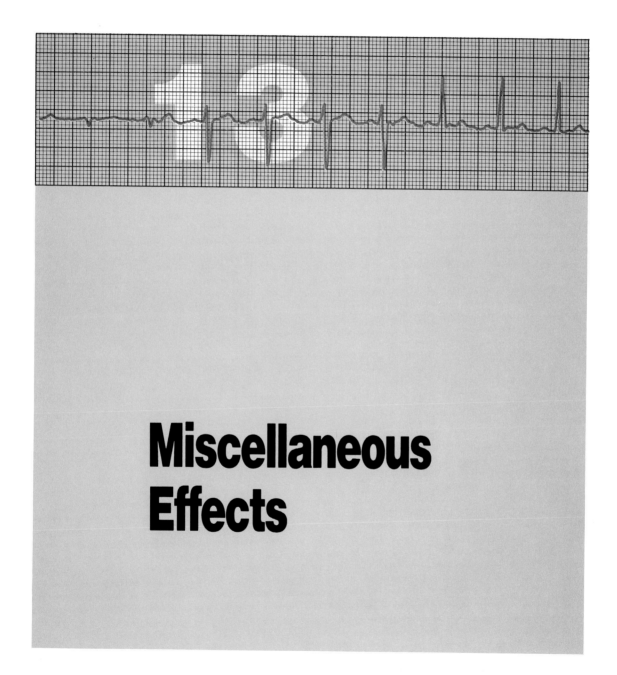

Miscellaneous Effects

This chapter discusses how ECGs may suggest electrolyte disturbances, demonstrate drug effects, pericarditis, dextrocardia, and early
repolarization; and an overview of pediatric ECGs is also included.

ELECTROLYTE DISTURBANCES

Electrolyte disturbances are only suggested on an ECG by ST-T abnormalities. In order to make a correct diagnosis, a clinical evaluation
must be correlated with the ECG results.

Hypokalemia. A lowered potassium concentration is suggested on an
ECG by a flat T wave and the occurrence of a U wave. ST depression
is sometimes present.

U WAVE

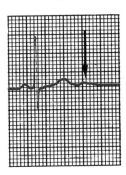

HYPOKALEMIA

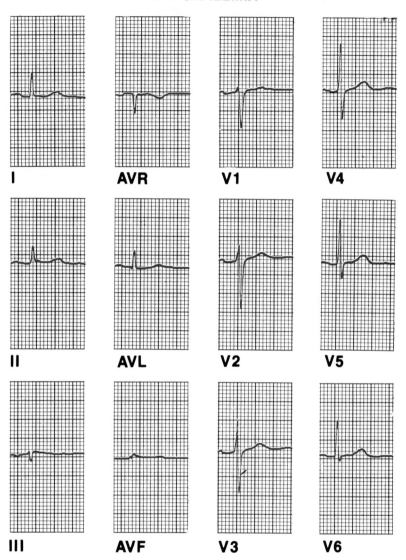

I AVR V1 V4

II AVL V2 V5

III AVF V3 V6

Hyperkalemia. An elevated serum potassium level is indicated on the ECG by peaked or tent-shaped T waves.

TENT-SHAPED T WAVE

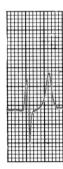

HYPERKALEMIA

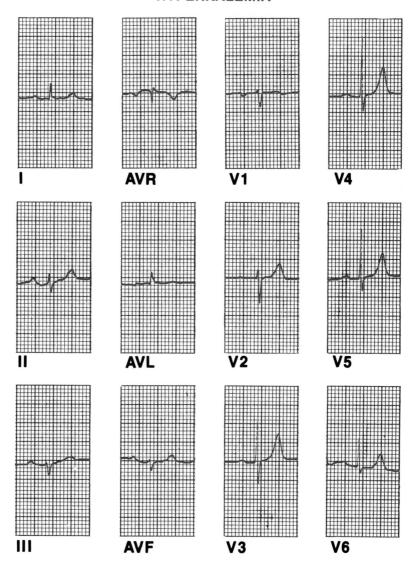

I AVR V1 V4

II AVL V2 V5

III AVF V3 V6

Hypocalcemia. A reduced calcium concentration is reflected on the ECG by a prolonged QT interval, which is a result of prolongation of the ST segment.

PROLONGED ST SEGMENT

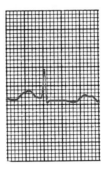

HYPOCALCEMIA

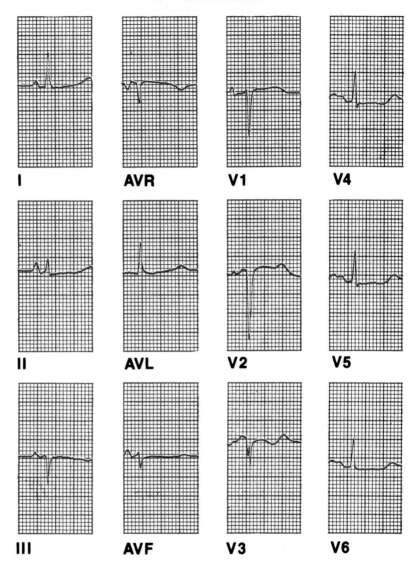

I AVR V1 V4

II AVL V2 V5

III AVF V3 V6

Hypercalcemia. An elevation of the serum calcium level is displayed on the ECG by a shortened QT interval, which is due to a short or absent ST segment.

SHORT ST SEGMENT

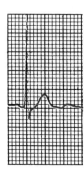

HYPERCALCEMIA

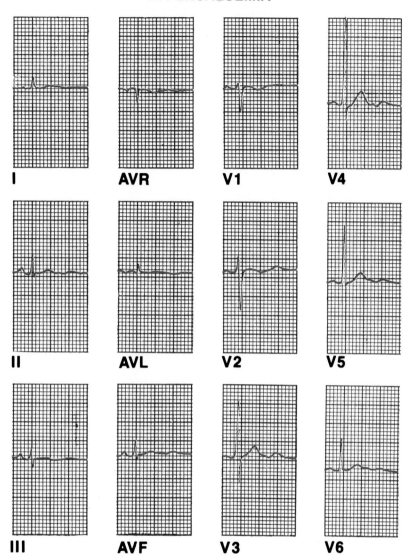

I   AVR   V1   V4

II   AVL   V2   V5

III   AVF   V3   V6

DRUG EFFECTS

Digitalis. Digitalis causes a characteristic downward sloping or scooping of the ST segment and a flattened or inverted T wave. The ST-T changes are usually seen in the leads with tall R waves, and these changes often mask ischemic changes.

ST SCOOPING

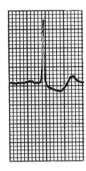

DIGITALIS EFFECT

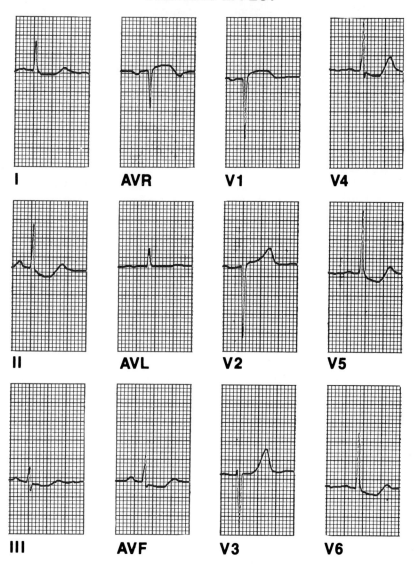

I   AVR   V1   V4

II   AVL   V2   V5

III   AVF   V3   V6

MISCELLANEOUS EFFECTS

Quinidine. The repolarization time of the ventricles is increased with the use of quinidine, producing a prolonged QT interval and ST-T abnormalities.

MARKED QT PROLONGATION

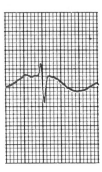

QUINIDINE EFFECT

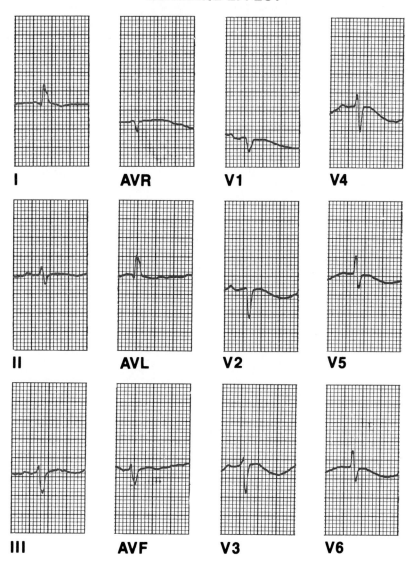

PERICARDITIS

Pericarditis is an inflammation of the pericardial sac surrounding the heart. The ECG demonstrates ST segment elevation, which assumes a concave curvature and subsequent T wave inversion.

PERICARDITIS

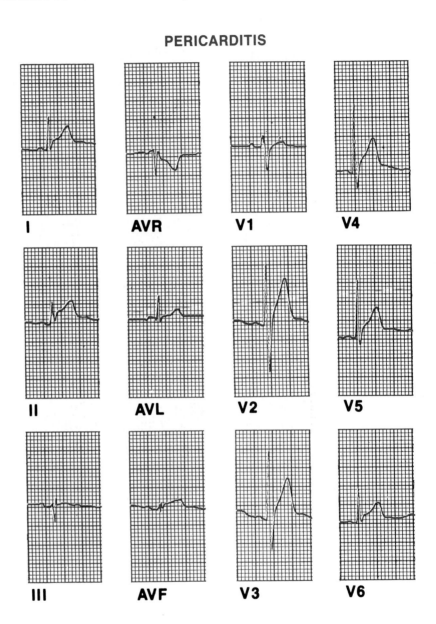

I AVR V1 V4

II AVL V2 V5

III AVF V3 V6

EARLY REPOLARIZATION

Early repolarization is characterized by ST segment elevation, especially in the left precordial leads—V$_4$, V$_5$, and V$_6$. The etiology for early repolarization is not entirely understood, but it is considered to be a normal variant.

EARLY REPOLARIZATION

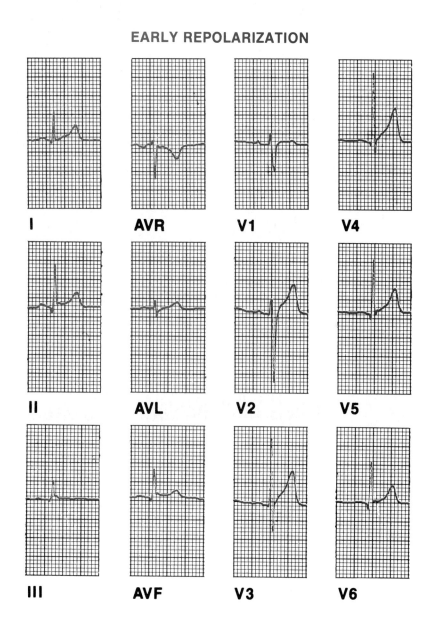

I	AVR	V1	V4
II	AVL	V2	V5
III	AVF	V3	V6

Making a distinction between pericarditis and early repolarization is best accomplished with the use of serial ECGs. The ST elevation of early repolarization remains unaffected by time, but the ST elevation of pericarditis eventually normalizes, and subsequent T wave inversion will often occur.

DEXTROCARDIA

Dextrocardia is demonstrated by complete transposition of the heart to the right side of the chest cavity. The ECG illustrates a mirror image of a normal ECG, resembling a tracing recorded with reversed arm leads and chest leads positioned on the wrong side of the chest cavity. The P, QRS, and T waves will be inverted in lead I and upright in aVR. R wave progression will be reversed and the tallest R wave will occur in V_1, which will be the lead nearest the heart, and as the chest leads move away from the heart a total loss of R waves will occur.

DEXTROCARDIA

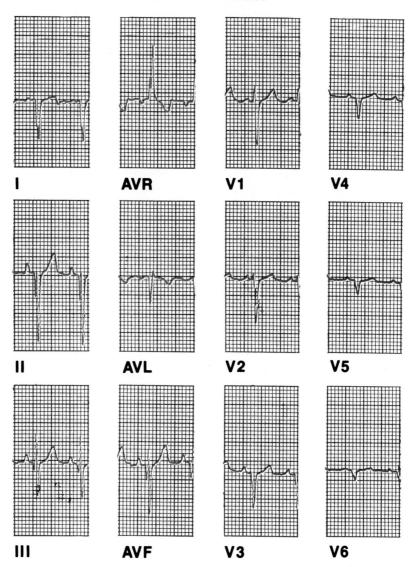

I AVR V1 V4

II AVL V2 V5

III AVF V3 V6

MISCELLANEOUS EFFECTS

PEDIATRIC ECGS

At birth, the right ventricle is as thick or thicker than the left, and the ECG demonstrates right ventricular hypertrophy. In utero, the resistance to flow in the systemic circulation is lower than in the pulmonary vascular bed, so the work of the right ventricle is much greater than that of the left. After birth, there is a decrease in right ventricular pressure and an increase in systemic resistance, and the left ventricle becomes thicker than the right.

Right axis deviation is also observed and may remain up to one year or more. T waves are normally inverted in V_1 through V_3, and are occasionally further leftward.

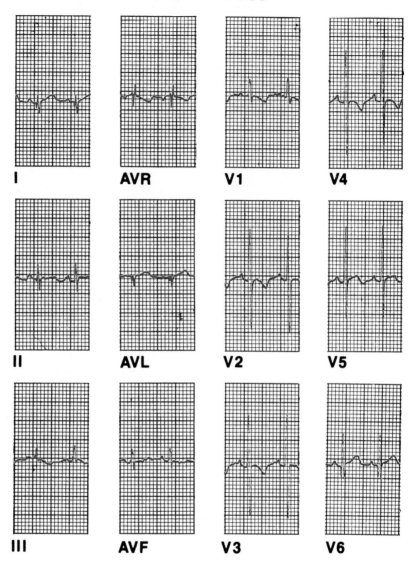

I   AVR   V1   V4

II   AVL   V2   V5

III   AVF   V3   V6

MISCELLANEOUS EFFECTS

HYPOKALEMIA

Check All ECG Leads for Hypokalemia

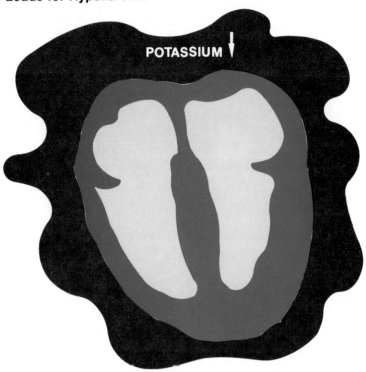

Criterion

Presence of a U wave and a flattened T wave

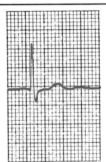

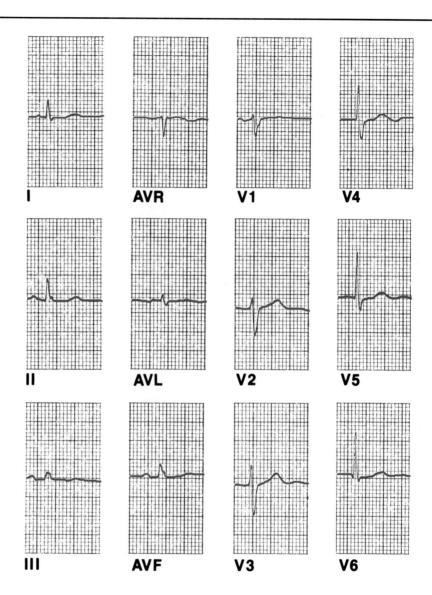

I	AVR	V1	V4
II	AVL	V2	V5
III	AVF	V3	V6

HYPERKALEMIA

Check All ECG Leads for Hyperkalemia

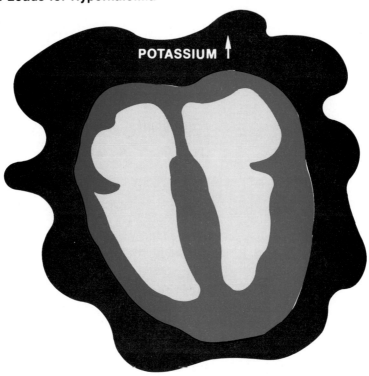

Criterion

Peaked and tent-shaped T waves

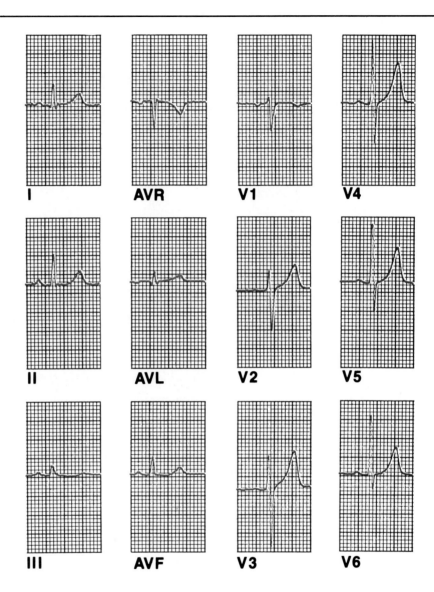

I	AVR	V1	V4
II	AVL	V2	V5
III	AVF	V3	V6

HYPOCALCEMIA

Check All ECG Leads for Hypocalcemia

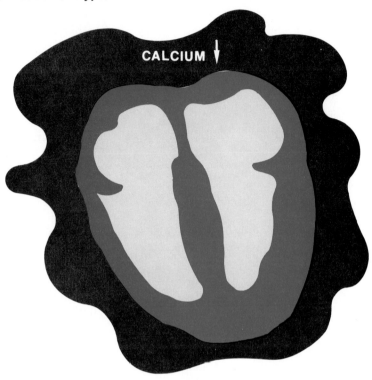

Criterion

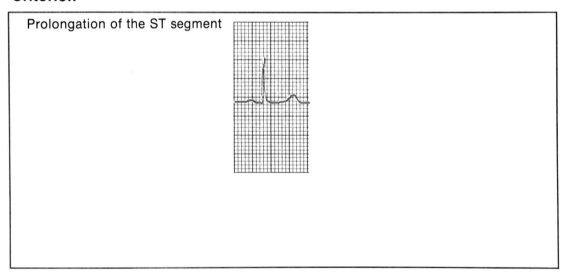

Prolongation of the ST segment

HOW TO QUICKLY AND ACCURATELY MASTER ECG INTERPRETATION

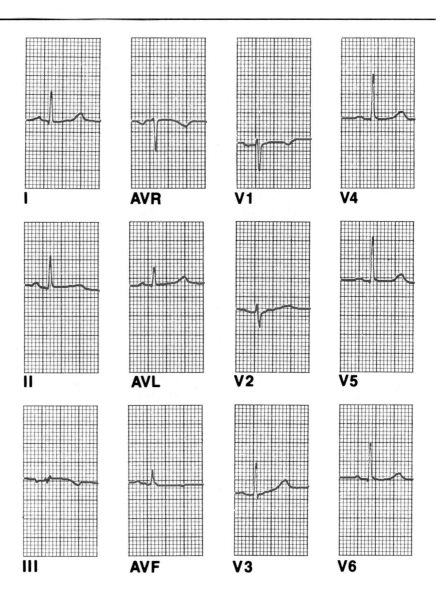

I AVR V1 V4

II AVL V2 V5

III AVF V3 V6

HYPERCALCEMIA

Check All ECG Leads for Hypercalcemia

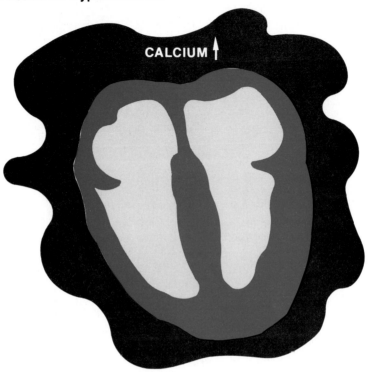

Criterion

Shortening of the ST segment

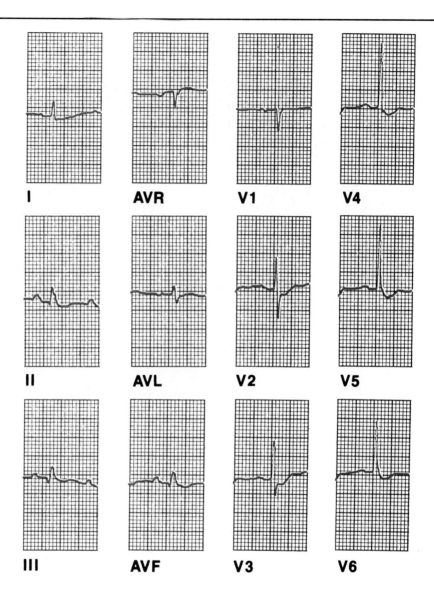

I AVR V1 V4

II AVL V2 V5

III AVF V3 V6

MISCELLANEOUS EFFECTS

241

DIGITALIS EFFECT

ECG Leads to Check for Digitalis Effect

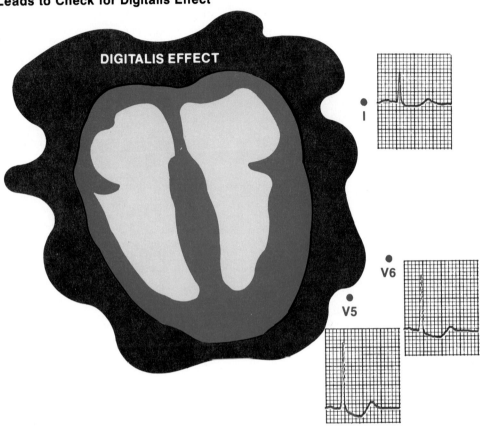

Criterion

Downward sloping or scooping of the ST segment and a flattened or inverted T wave, best seen in leads with tall R waves

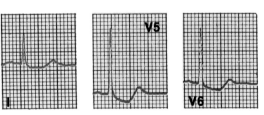

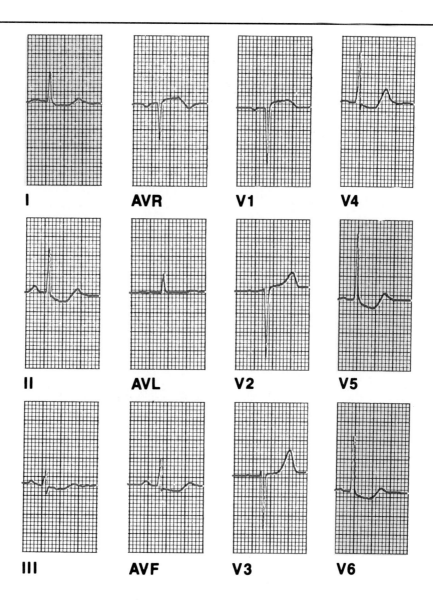

I AVR V1 V4

II AVL V2 V5

III AVF V3 V6

MISCELLANEOUS EFFECTS

QUINIDINE EFFECT

Check All ECG Leads for Quinidine Effect

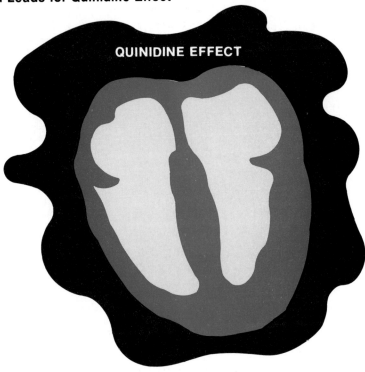

QUINIDINE EFFECT

Criterion

Prolonged QT interval and ST-T abnormalities

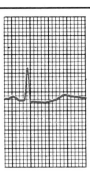

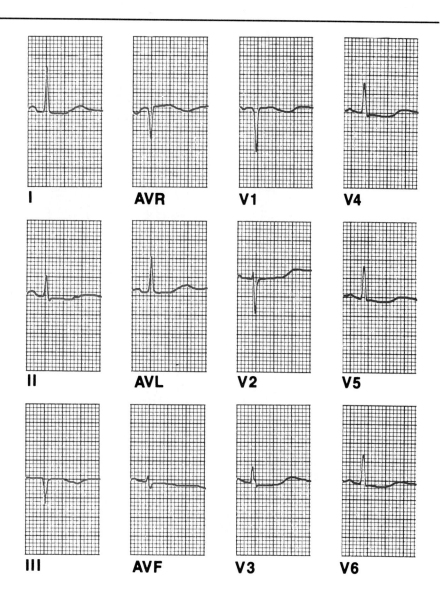

I   AVR   V1   V4

II   AVL   V2   V5

III   AVF   V3   V6

MISCELLANEOUS EFFECTS

PERICARDITIS

Check All ECG Leads for Pericarditis

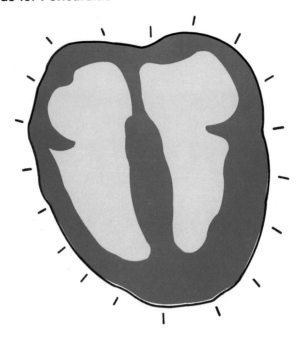

Criterion

ST segment elevation that assumes a concave curvature

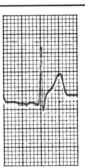

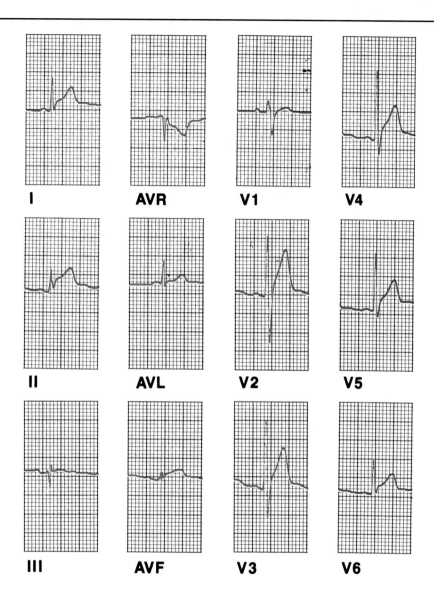

I	AVR	V1	V4
II	AVL	V2	V5
III	AVF	V3	V6

EARLY REPOLARIZATION

ECG Leads to Check for Early Repolarization

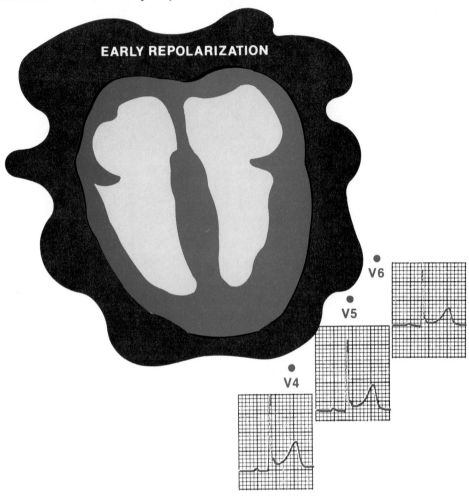

EARLY REPOLARIZATION

V6

V5

V4

Criterion

ST segment elevation, especially in V_4, V_5, and V_6

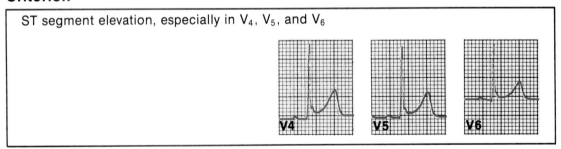

V4   V5   V6

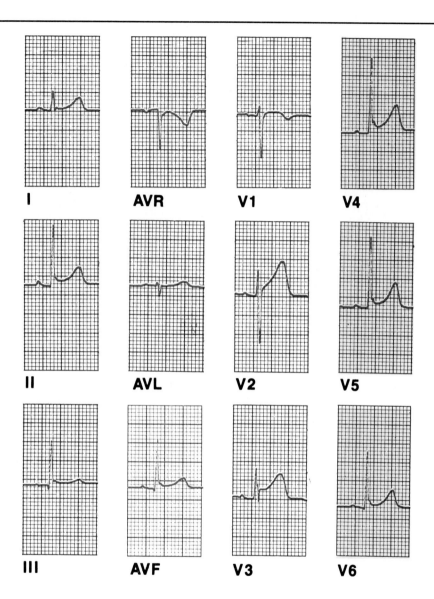

I AVR V1 V4

II AVL V2 V5

III AVF V3 V6

DEXTROCARDIA

ECG Leads to Check for Dextrocardia

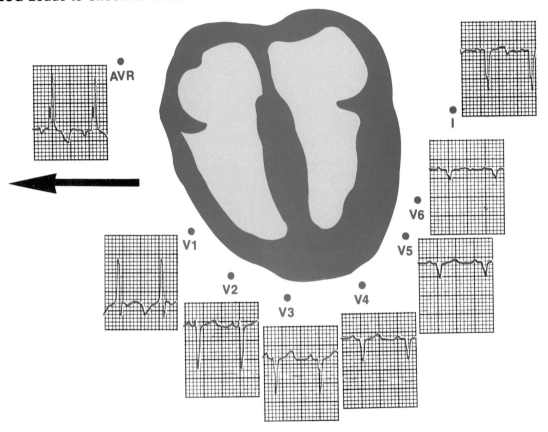

Criteria

1. P, QRS, and T waves often inverted in lead I

2. P, QRS, and T waves upright in aVR

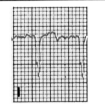 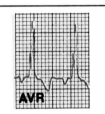

3. R wave progression will be reversed—the tallest R wave occurs in V_1 and will become progressively smaller as the chest leads move away from the heart.

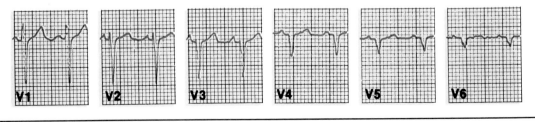

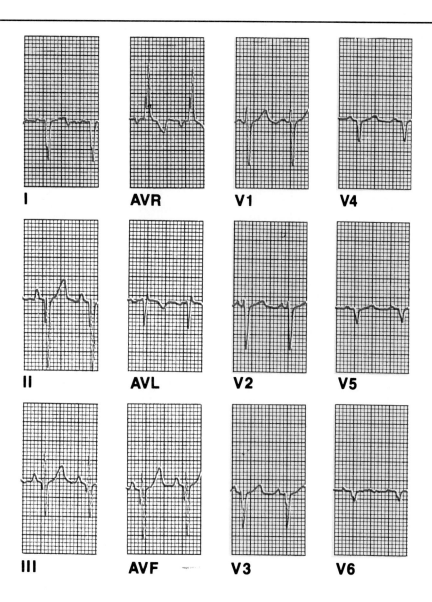

I AVR V1 V4

II AVL V2 V5

III AVF V3 V6

PEDIATRIC ECGS

ECG Leads to Check for Pediatric ECG

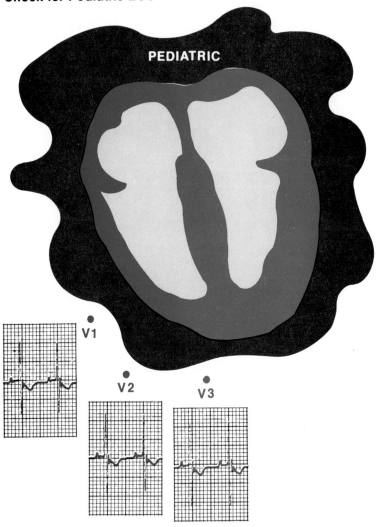

Criteria

1. Right axis deviation is present.

2. T waves may be inverted in V_1, V_2, and V_3.

3. Sinus tachycardia is a normal manifestation in infancy.

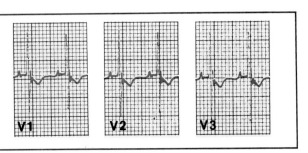

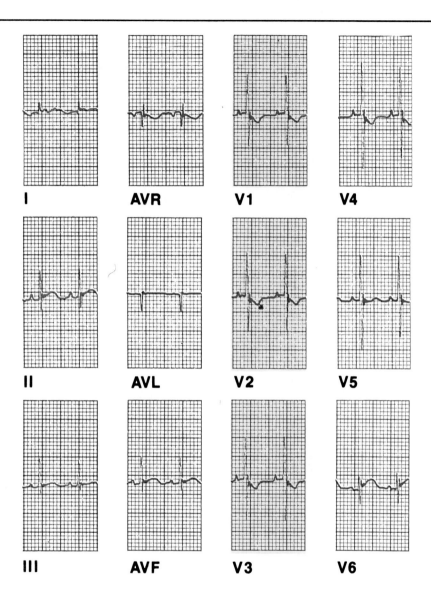

I   AVR   V1   V4

II   AVL   V2   V5

III   AVF   V3   V6

MISCELLANEOUS EFFECTS

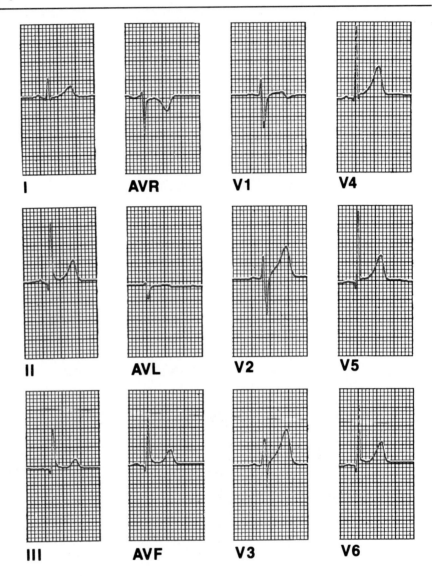

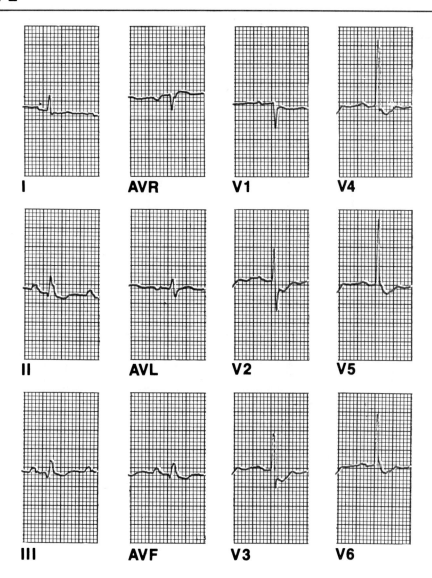

I AVR V1 V4

II AVL V2 V5

III AVF V3 V6

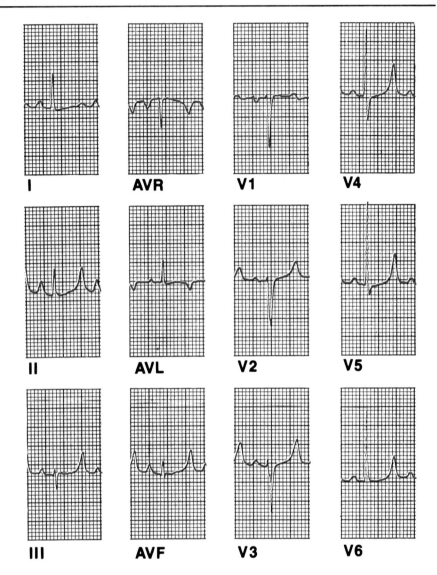

I AVR V1 V4

II AVL V2 V5

III AVF V3 V6

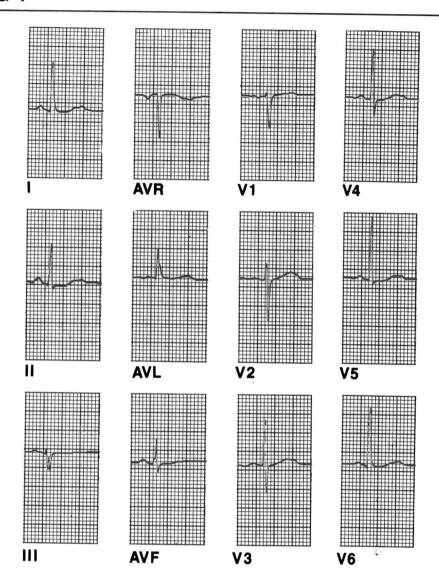

I AVR V1 V4

II AVL V2 V5

III AVF V3 V6

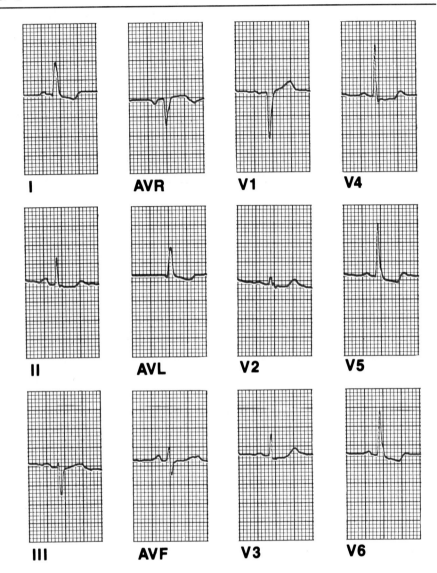

I   AVR   V1   V4

II   AVL   V2   V5

III   AVF   V3   V6

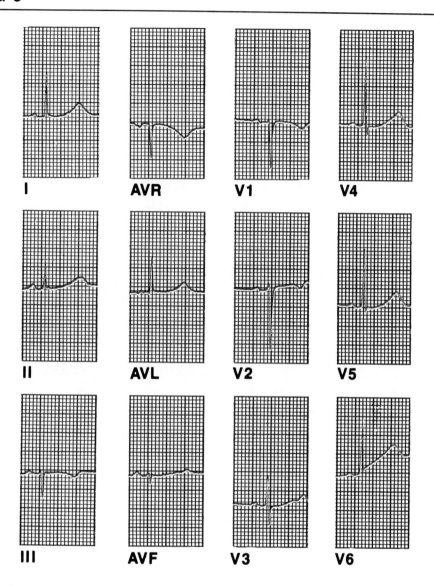

I AVR V1 V4

II AVL V2 V5

III AVF V3 V6

MISCELLANEOUS EFFECTS

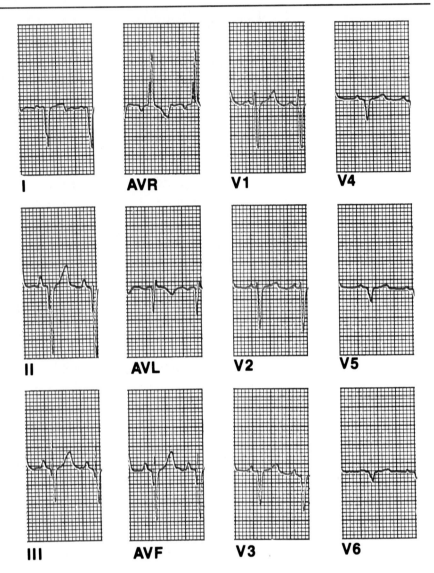

I   AVR   V1   V4

II   AVL   V2   V5

III   AVF   V3   V6

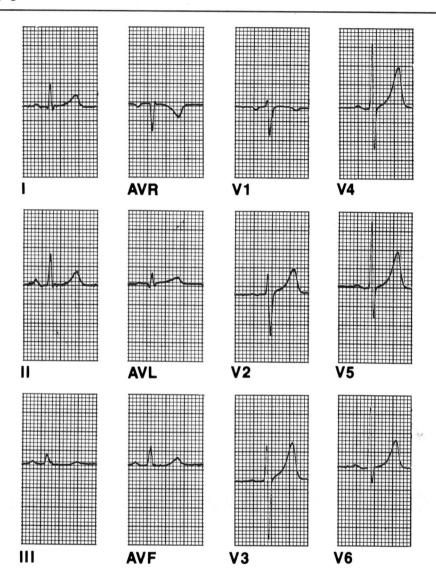

I AVR V1 V4

II AVL V2 V5

III AVF V3 V6

MISCELLANEOUS EFFECTS

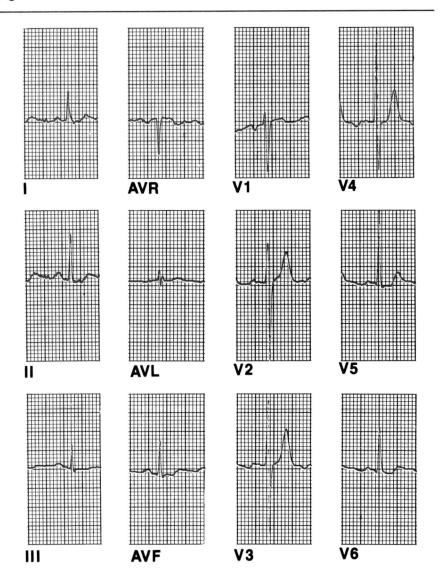

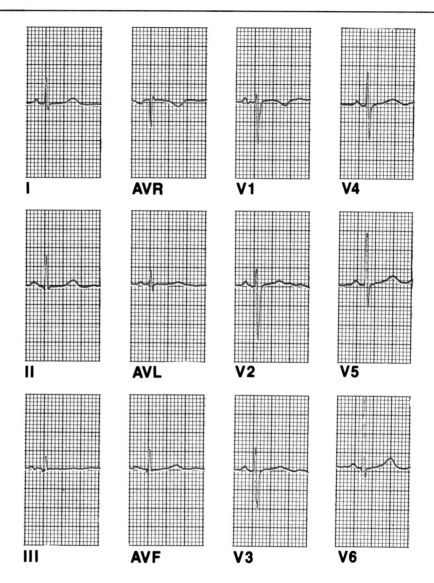

I AVR V1 V4

II AVL V2 V5

III AVF V3 V6

MISCELLANEOUS EFFECTS

REVIEW ECG ANSWERS

1. Early repolarization vs. pericarditis
2. Hypercalcemia
3. Right atrial hypertrophy, hyperkalemia, and hypocalcemia
4. Hypokalemia
5. Digitalis effect
6. Hypocalcemia
7. Dextrocardia
8. Hyperkalemia
9. Hyperkalemia
10. Hypokalemia

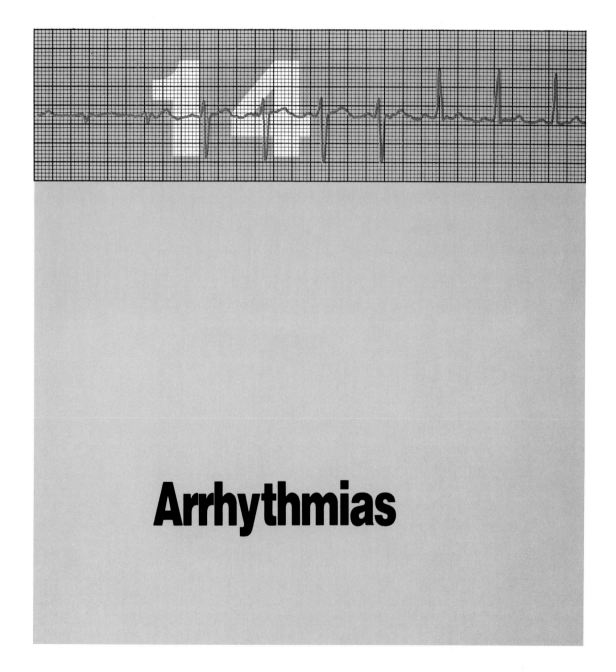

Arrhythmias

This chapter is not meant to be an exhaustive study on the subject of abnormal rhythms, but rather an introduction to basic arrhythmias and a list of criteria for each abnormality. Many other arrhythmia books are available for a more intensive study.

A schematic view of the heart will be used throughout this section to illustrate the electrical conduction system and to demonstrate impulse formation and the conduction pathways used for each arrhythmia. Each arrhythmia will be presented with a diagram of the electrical conduction system with the respective abnormality depicted, a list of criteria, and an ECG representation.

BASIC CONCEPTS

Although the sinus node is the pacemaker of the heart, there are other potential pacemaker sites:

Atria
AV node
Ventricles

POTENTIAL PACEMAKER SITES

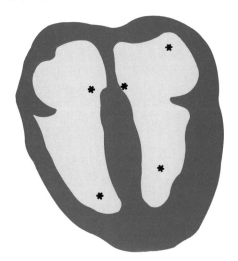

The following criteria are used for recognition of an APC:

1. It occurs early in the cardiac cycle.
2. The ectopic P wave differs in configuration from the sinus P wave because the atria are depolarized from a different direction.
3. QRS usually resembles QRS in the normal cardiac cycle.

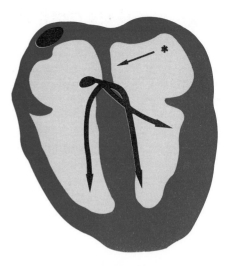

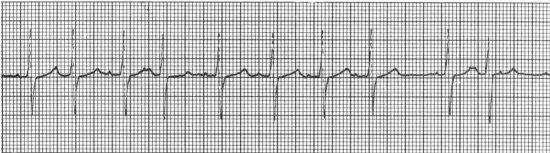

Sinus Tachycardia With Isolated APCs

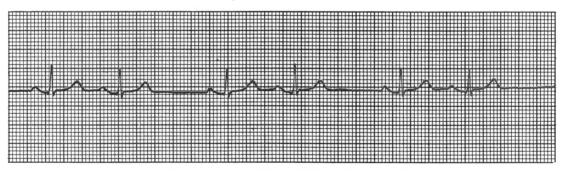

Sinus Rhythm With APCs in Bigeminy

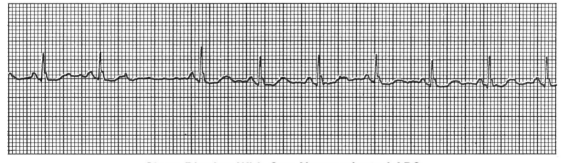

Sinus Rhythm With One Nonconducted APC

JUNCTIONAL PREMATURE CONTRACTIONS

Junctional or nodal premature contractions (JPCs or NPCs) are early ectopic beats that begin in the AV node or junctional tissue surrounding the AV node.

An early impulse travels forward through the normal conduction pathways, inscribing a normal QRS. Simultaneously, the impulse moves retrogradely to depolarize the atria. A negative P wave is recorded because the atria are depolarized from a backward direction.

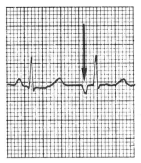 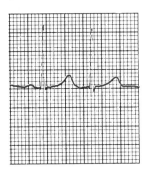 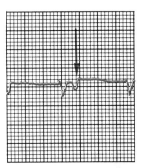

JPC With Inverted P Wave Preceding QRS

JPC With No P Wave Visible

JPC With Inverted P Wave Following QRS

JPCs may be isolated or may occur up to six in a row. Six or more JPCs in a row constitute a junctional tachycardia.

As with APCs, JPCs may also be nonconducted. An early inverted P wave is found in or immediately after the preceding T wave, and is not followed by a QRS complex.

The following criteria are used for recognition of a JPC:

1. It occurs early in the cardiac cycle.
2. A negative P wave precedes QRS with a PR interval shorter than the PR interval of dominant rhythm. The retrograde conduction to the atria is faster than the antegrade conduction to the ventricles.

   No P wave precedes QRS. The P wave is buried in the QRS complex because antegrade conduction to the ventricles and retrograde conduction to the atria occur simultaneously.

   Negative P wave follows QRS. Antegrade conduction to the ventricles is faster than retrograde conduction to the atria.
3. QRS usually resembles QRS in the normal cardiac cycle.

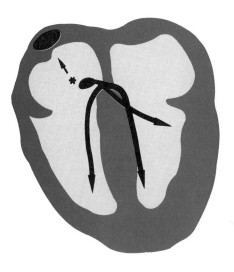

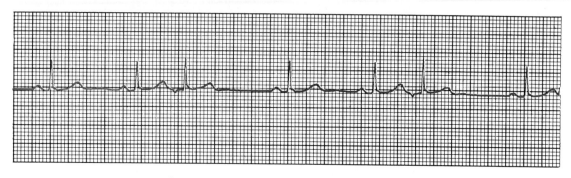

Sinus Rhythm With JPCs in Trigeminy

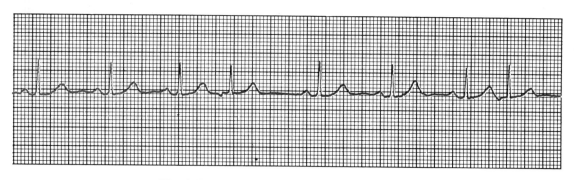

Sinus Rhythm With JPCs in Quadrigeminy

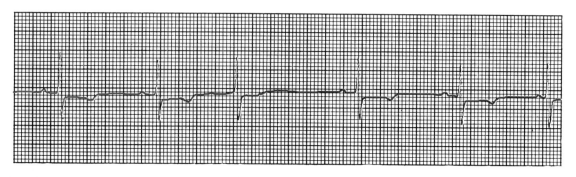

Sinus Rhythm With Isolated JPC

VENTRICULAR PREMATURE CONTRACTIONS

Ventricular premature contractions (VPCs) are early ectopic beats that begin in the ventricles. An early impulse begins in one ventricle and spreads to the other with some delay because of slow conduction through ventricular muscle. This slow spread of conduction causes a widened QRS complex. The ventricles depolarize first, inscribing a widened QRS, while the atrial cycle continues independently, uninterrupted by the VPC.

End diastolic VPC. A VPC that occurs immediately after the atria have depolarized from a sinus impulse is an *end diastolic* VPC. A sinus P wave is either partially or completely inscribed, followed immediately by a VPC. The sinus P wave has no connection with the VPC. Each has occurred independently and almost concurrently.

SINUS P WAVE

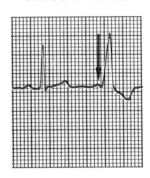

End Diastolic VPC

Interpolated VPC. A VPC that is sandwiched between two consecutive sinus beats with no pause following it is an *interpolated* VPC.

SINUS P WAVES

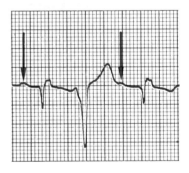

Interpolated VPC

Malignant VPC. A VPC that falls on the T wave of the previous beat and makes the heart vulnerable to the possibility of repetitive firing of the ventricular focus is a *malignant* VPC.

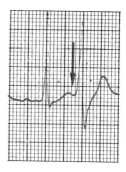

Malignant VPC

VPCs may be isolated or may occur up to six in a row. Six or more VPCs in a row constitute a ventricular tachycardia.

The following criteria are used for recognition of a VPC:

1. It occurs early in the cardiac cycle.
2. No ectopic P wave is present. Although the sinus P wave may occur either directly before or after the QRS, it bears no relationship to it.
3. QRS is wide and bizarre (.12 second or greater) because conduction through ventricular myocardium is slower than through normal conduction pathways.

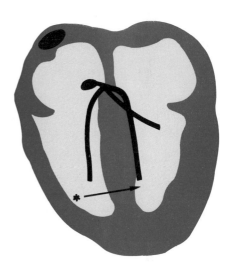

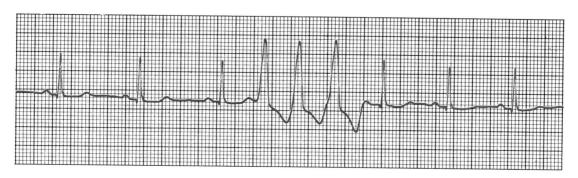

Sinus Rhythm With 3 Unifocal VPCs in a Row

ARRHYTHMIAS

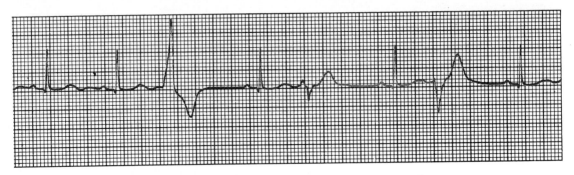

Sinus Rhythm With 3 Isolated Multifocal VPCs

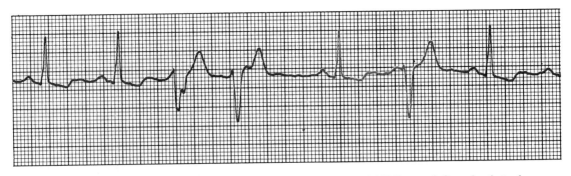

Sinus Rhythm With 3 Multifocal VPCs—One Pair of VPCs and One Isolated

ESCAPE BEATS

Escape beats are always late in relation to the dominant cardiac rhythm. When the dominant pacemaker does not fire, the escape mechanism fires and rescues the heart from asystole.

Escape beats may be isolated or may occur up to six in a row. Six or more escape beats in a row constitute an escape rhythm.

The following criteria are used for recognition of an AV junctional escape beat:

1. It is late in relation to the dominant cardiac rhythm.
2. It is preceded by either an inverted P wave, no P wave, or a sinus P wave with a short PR interval.
3. QRS is usually of normal duration.

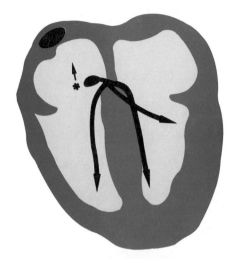

The following criteria are used for recognition of a ventricular escape beat:

1. It is late in relation to the dominant cardiac rhythm.
2. QRS is wide and bizarre.

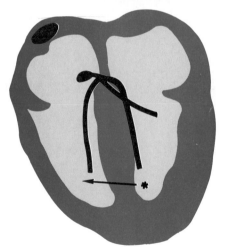

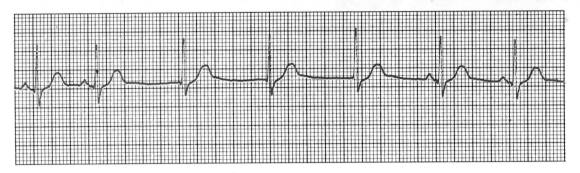

Sinus Rhythm With 3 Junctional Escape Beats

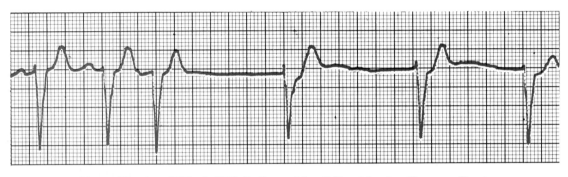

Sinus Rhythm With 1 APC Followed by 3 Ventricular Escape Beats

HOW TO QUICKLY AND ACCURATELY MASTER ECG INTERPRETATION

ATRIAL TACHYCARDIA

A run of six or more APCs in a row, usually between the rates of 140 to 220 beats per minute, determines an atrial tachycardia. Often the term *paroxysmal atrial tachycardia* (PAT) is used, meaning a sudden burst of unifocal APCs.

If the burst of atrial tachycardia is slower than 180 beats per minute, probably all the atrial impulses will conduct through the AV node to the ventricles. If the rate is faster, some of the impulses may find the AV node to be refractory from the previous beat, and all the ectopic P waves will not be conducted through the AV node to the ventricles. This is called *PAT with block*.

The following criteria are used for recognition of PAT:

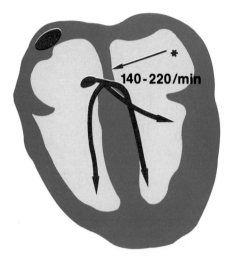

1. The first beat of rhythm is early.
2. Ectopic P waves are different in configuration from sinus P waves.
3. QRS usually resembles QRS of dominant rhythm.
4. The PR interval is constant.
5. The ventricular rate is 140 to 220 beats per minute.

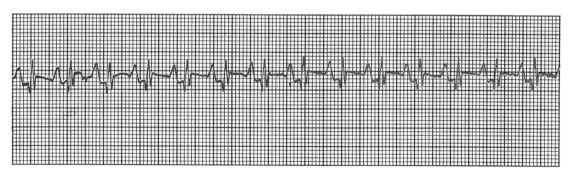

Atrial Tachycardia

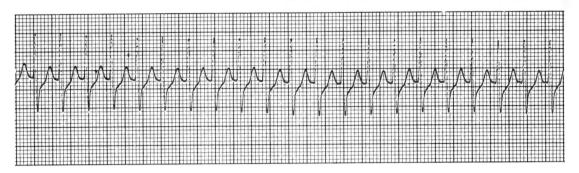

Atrial Tachycardia

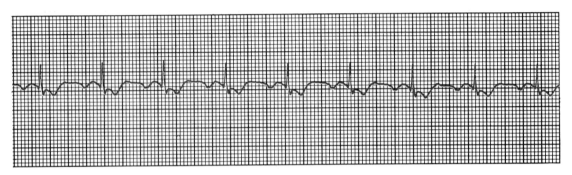

PAT With 2:1 Block—2 P Waves for Each QRS

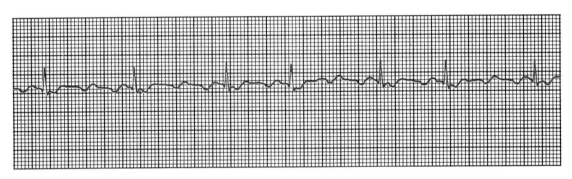

PAT With Varying Block—2 or 3 P Waves for Each QRS

MULTIFOCAL ATRIAL TACHYCARDIA

This arrhythmia is also called *chaotic atrial rhythm,* and is caused by the rapid and repetitive firing of two or more ectopic atrial foci. The rate is usually between 100 and 200 beats per minute. The ectopic impulses spread through the atria in an abnormal way, causing P waves to be different in configuration from the sinus P waves. Some of the ectopic P waves may be nonconducted.

The following criteria are used for recognition of multifocal atrial tachycardia:

1. There are multifocal early ectopic P waves with an irregular P-P cycle.
2. The PR interval varies from one beat to another.
3. Nonconducted ectopic P waves may occur.
4. QRS usually resembles QRS of dominant rhythm.
5. Atrial rate is 100 to 200 beats per minute.

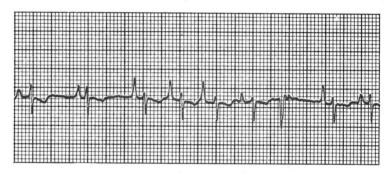

Varying P Waves and PR Intervals

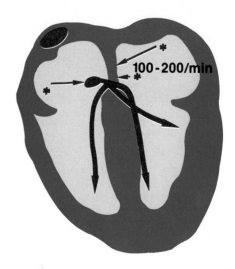

100-200/min

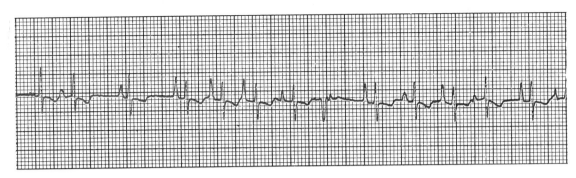

Multifocal Atrial Tachycardia

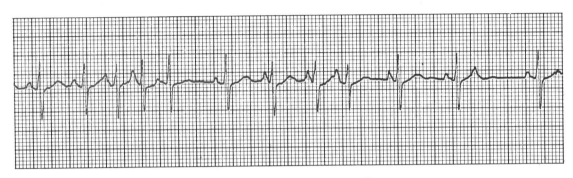

Multifocal Atrial Tachycardia

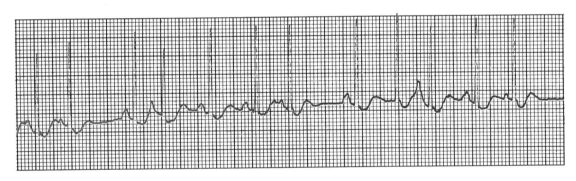

Multifocal Atrial Tachycardia

HOW TO QUICKLY AND ACCURATELY MASTER ECG INTERPRETATION

ATRIAL FLUTTER

One theory of impulse formation in atrial flutter is a rapid and repetitive firing of a unifocal atrial focus at a rate between 220 and 350 beats per minute. F waves replace P waves and take on a sawtooth configuration. Because the flutter waves occur so rapidly, it is difficult for the AV node to conduct all the impulses to the ventricles. The ventricles usually respond to the even-numbered waves—second, fourth, sixth, etc.—or may respond sporadically at various conduction ratios.

The following criteria are used for recognition of atrial flutter:

1. F waves replace P waves at a rate of 220 to 350 beats per minute.
2. The ventricular response is regular if the conduction ratio is constant, and irregular if the conduction ratio is variable.
3. QRS usually resembles QRS of dominant rhythm.

FLUTTER WAVES

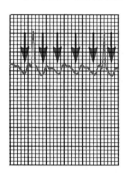

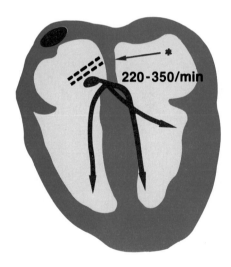

220-350/min

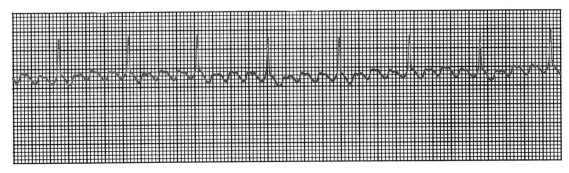

Atrial Flutter With 4:1 Block—4 F Waves for Each QRS

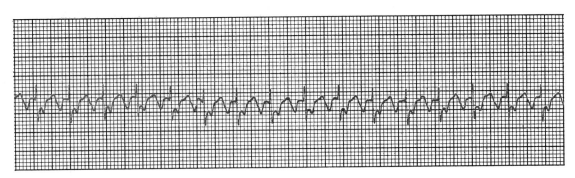

Atrial Flutter With 2:1 Block

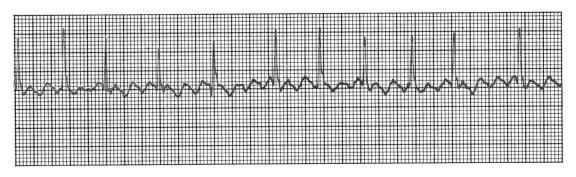

Atrial Flutter With Varying Conduction

ATRIAL FIBRILLATION

One theory of impulse formation in atrial fibrillation is that a rapid and repetitive firing of multifocal atrial ectopic foci occurs, at a rate of 350 to 650 beats per minute. One ectopic focus fires immediately after another, causing the atria to quiver continuously rather than contract. These fibrillatory or f waves' occurring so rapidly make it difficult to determine the atrial rate. f waves are divided into two categories, *coarse* and *fine.*

FIBRILLATORY WAVES

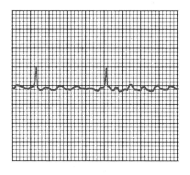

Coarse   **Fine**

Only some of the f waves are able to be intermittently conducted through the AV node to the ventricles because the AV node is constantly rendered refractory by the multitude of fibrillatory impulses, causing a very irregular ventricular rate.

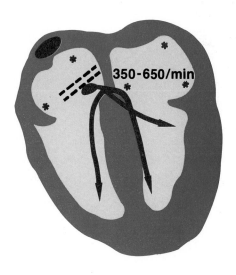

The following criteria are used for recognition of atrial fibrillation:

1. Multifocal f waves replace P waves at a rate of 350 to 650 beats per minute.
2. Irregularly irregular ventricular response (R-R cycle constantly varies).
3. QRS usually resembles QRS of dominant rhythm.

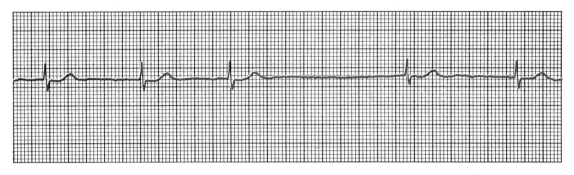

Atrial Fibrillation

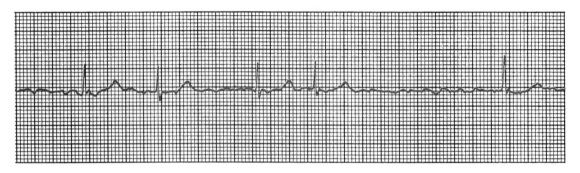

Atrial Fibrillation

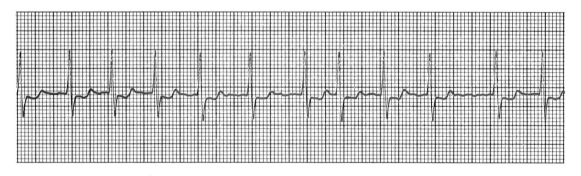

Atrial Fibrillation

JUNCTIONAL ESCAPE RHYTHM

A junctional or idionodal escape rhythm is a run of six or more junctional escape beats at a rate of 40 to 60 beats per minute. This mechanism takes over as the heart rhythm when the sinus node fails to fire or when there is a blockage in the conduction system.

The following criteria are used for recognition of a junctional escape rhythm:

1. The first beat of the escape rhythm is a late beat.
2. A negative ectopic P wave either precedes or follows the QRS, no P wave is discernible; or a sinus P wave precedes the QRS with a shortened PR interval, indicating lack of conduction.
3. QRS usually resembles QRS of dominant rhythm.
4. The rate is usually 40 to 60 beats per minute.

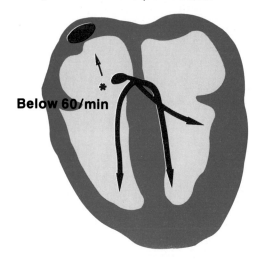

Below 60/min

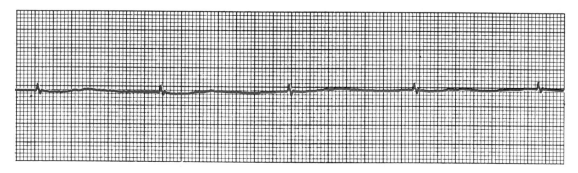

Junctional Escape Rhythm

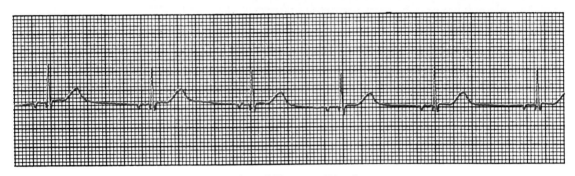

Junctional Escape Rhythm

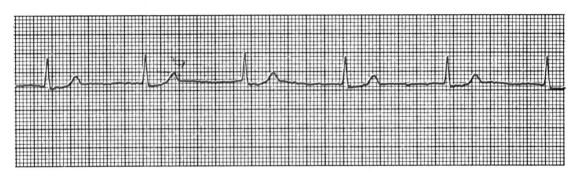

Junctional Escape Rhythm

JUNCTIONAL AND ACCELERATED
JUNCTIONAL TACHYCARDIA

Rapid and repetitive firing of six or more JPCs in a row constitutes a junctional or accelerated junctional tachycardia.

The following criteria are used for recognition of junctional and accelerated junctional tachycardia:

1. An early negative P wave either precedes or follows QRS, or no P wave is discernible.
2. QRS usually resembles QRS of dominant rhythm.
3. The junctional tachycardia rate is 60 to 160 beats per minute. The accelerated junctional tachycardia rate is 160 to 220 beats per minute.

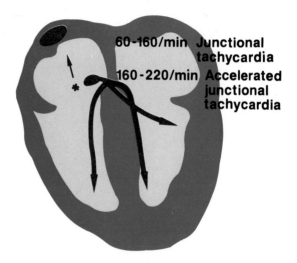

60-160/min Junctional tachycardia

160-220/min Accelerated junctional tachycardia

When you are unable to differentiate between an atrial and a junctional tachycardia, the term *supraventricular tachycardia* is used, denoting a tachycardia with a focus located somewhere above the ventricles.

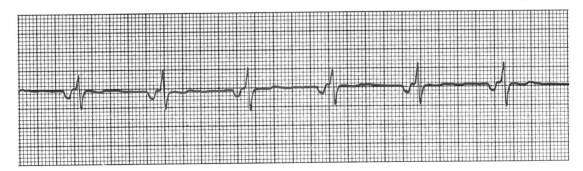

Junctional Tachycardia

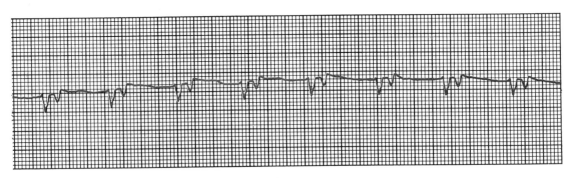

Junctional Tachycardia

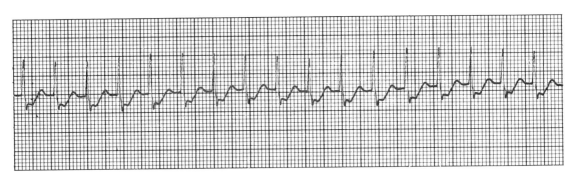

Accelerated Junctional Tachycardia

VENTRICULAR ESCAPE RHYTHM AND ACCELERATED IDIOVENTRICULAR RHYTHM

Ventricular escape or idioventricular escape rhythm is a repetitive firing of six or more ventricular escape beats at an inherent rate of 40 beats per minute or less. This mechanism takes over as the heart rhythm when the sinus node fails to fire or when there is a blockage in the conduction system.

The following criteria are used for recognition of ventricular escape rhythm:

1. The first beat of escape rhythm is a late beat.
2. No ectopic P waves are present.
3. QRS complex is wide and bizarre.
4. The rate is 40 beats per minute or less.

An accelerated idioventricular rhythm is a repetitive firing of six or more VPCs at a rate of 40 to 100 beats per minute.

The following criteria are used for recognition of an accelerated idioventricular rhythm:

1. No ectopic P waves are present.
2. QRS complex is wide and bizarre.
3. The rate is 40 to 100 beats per minute.

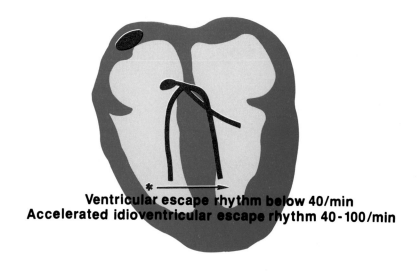

Ventricular escape rhythm below 40/min
Accelerated idioventricular escape rhythm 40-100/min

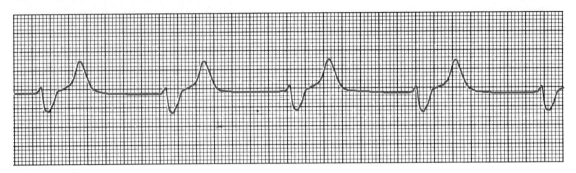

Ventricular Escape Rhythm

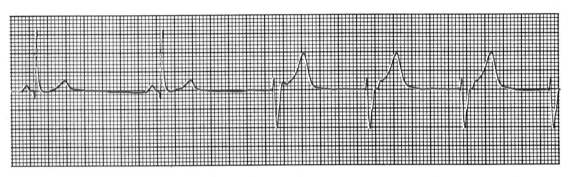

Sinus Bradycardia Followed by a Run of Accelerated Idioventricular Rhythm

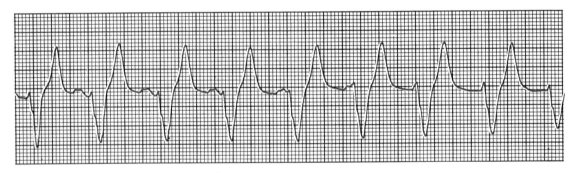

Accelerated Idioventricular Rhythm

VENTRICULAR TACHYCARDIA

Ventricular tachycardia is a rapid and repetitive firing of six or more VPCs in a row. When the ventricles depolarize and contract rapidly, the volume of blood ejected into the systemic circulation is often inadequate.

The following criteria are used for recognition of ventricular tachycardia:

1. The first beat of rhythm is early.
2. No ectopic P waves are present. If the heart rhythm is sinus, the sinus P waves usually continue unaffected by the tachycardia.
3. QRS complex is wide and bizarre.
4. The rate is between 100 and 250 beats per minute.

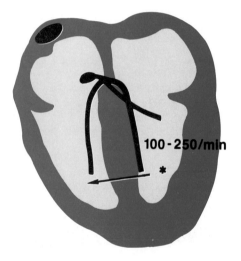

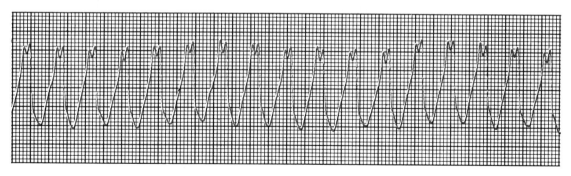

Ventricular Tachycardia

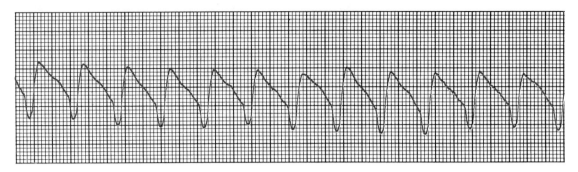

Ventricular Tachycardia

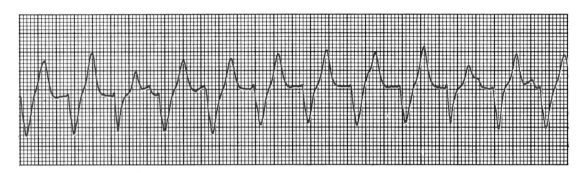

Ventricular Tachycardia

VENTRICULAR FLUTTER AND VENTRICULAR FIBRILLATION

Ventricular flutter is a rapid and repetitive firing of one or more ventricular ectopic foci at a rate of 150 to 300 beats per minute with a fairly regular rhythm.

The following criteria are used for recognition of ventricular flutter:

1. No atrial activity can be recognized.
2. QRS complexes appear to run into each other with no visible ST segments or T waves.
3. The ventricular rate is 150 to 300 beats per minute.

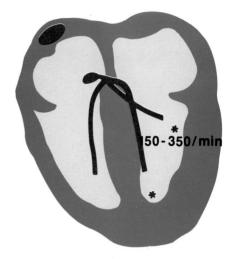

Ventricular fibrillation is a rapid and repetitive firing of multifocal ventricular ectopic foci in an irregular fashion with a rate of 150 to 500 beats per minute. Virtually no blood is ejected into the systemic circulation.

The following criteria are used for recognition of ventricular fibrillation:

1. No atrial activity can be recognized.
2. No QRS complexes can be recognized.
3. The rhythm is very irregular and is 150 to 500 beats per minute.

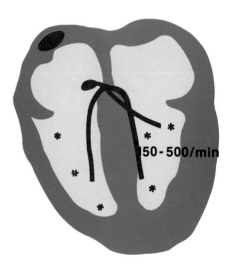

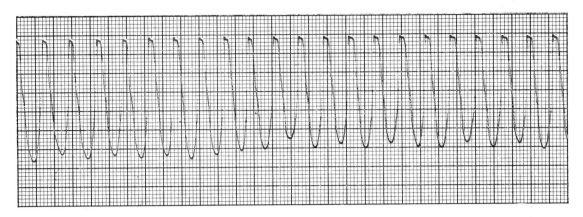

Ventricular Flutter

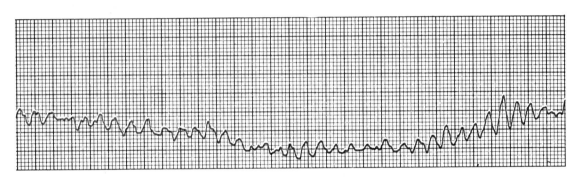

Ventricular Fibrillation

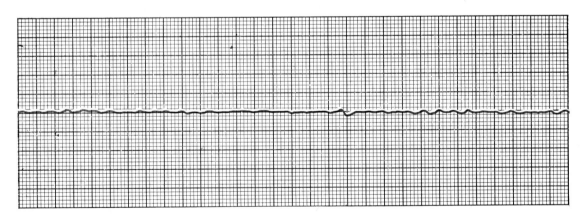

Ventricular Fibrillation

HOW TO QUICKLY AND ACCURATELY MASTER ECG INTERPRETATION

AV DISSOCIATION

AV dissociation is a double rhythm in which the atria and ventricles beat independently, each under the control of a separate pacemaking focus.

The atrial focus depolarizes the atria and either an ectopic focus in the AV node or the ventricles take over the business of depolarizing the ventricles. If the atria are in sinus rhythm, the P wave floats in and out of the QRS complex, but usually bears no relationship to it.

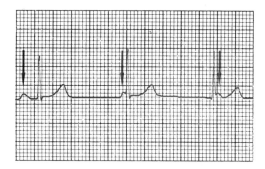

P Wave Floats in and out of QRS Complex

The following criteria are used for recognition of AV dissociation:

1. With the atria in sinus rhythm, there is one P wave for each QRS complex, but it usually bears no relationship to it. The P waves float in and out of the QRS and occasionally conduct to the ventricles.
2. The ventricles are under the control of either an AV junctional or ventricular focus.

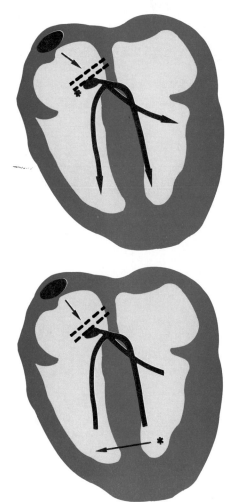

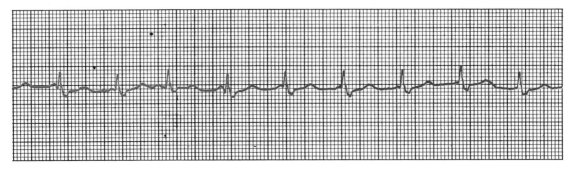

AV Dissociation Between Sinus Rhythm and Junctional Tachycardia

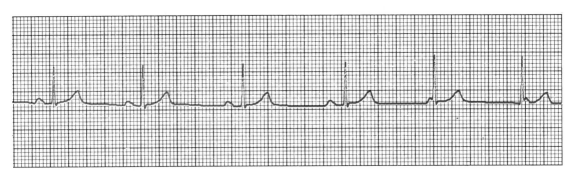

AV Dissociation Between Sinus Bradycardia and Junctional Escape Rhythm

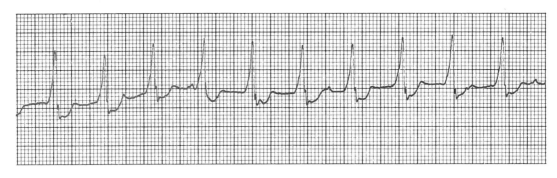

AV Dissociation Between Sinus Rhythm and Ventricular Tachycardia

ABERRATION

Aberration is a variation or change in the QRS complex from the normal configuration, and it occurs when a sinus or supraventricular impulse activates the ventricles in an abnormal way. The impulse travels down the conduction pathways and finds one of the bundle branches to be refractory from the previous beat, so conduction takes place abnormally from one ventricle to another, through ventricular myocardium. Because of the delay in conduction, a wide and bizarre QRS complex results.

Two causes of aberration are as follows:

1. APCs or JPCs occur so close to the previous beat that one of the bundle branches is still refractory.
2. During irregular ventricular rates when a long R-R cycle takes place, the refractory period of the bundle branches normally lengthens, and if the next R-R cycle is shorter it may find one of the bundle branches to be refractory, and aberration will occur. This type of aberration is called the *Ashman phenomenon* and is often found in atrial fibrillation.

EARLY P WAVE   **INVERTED EARLY P WAVE**   **LONG R-R FOLLOWED BY SHORT R-R CYCLE**

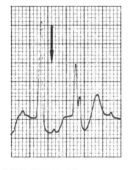
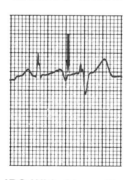
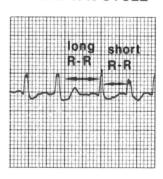

APC With Aberration   **JPC With Aberration**   **Atrial Fibrillation With Aberration**

The following criteria are used for recognition of aberration:

1. An APC with aberration is recognized by an early ectopic P wave preceding a wide and bizarre QRS.
2. A JPC with aberration is recognized by an inverted early ectopic P wave either preceding or immediately following a wide and bizarre QRS.
3. Atrial fibrillation with aberration is recognized by a long R-R cycle followed by a short R-R cycle, followed in turn by a wide and bizarre QRS.

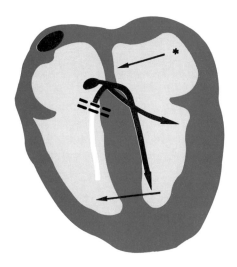

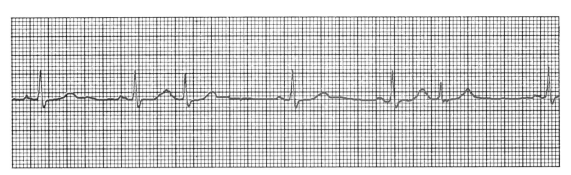

APCs With Aberration in Trigeminy

HOW TO QUICKLY AND ACCURATELY MASTER ECG INTERPRETATION

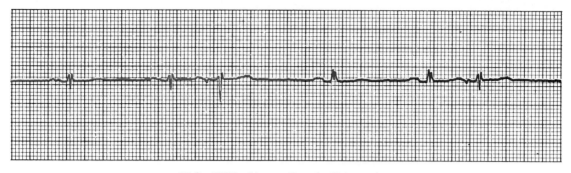

JPCs With Aberration in Trigeminy

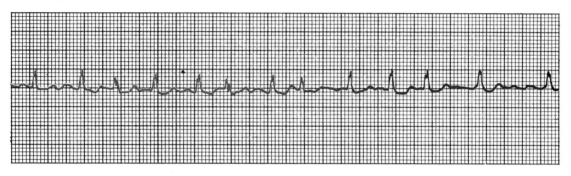

Atrial Fibrillation With Aberrancy

SECOND DEGREE AV BLOCK WENCKEBACH

When the conduction of sinus or supraventricular impulses is delayed or interrupted at the AV junction, AV block is said to be present. When we discuss nonconducted APCs, atrial flutter with varying conduction, PAT with block, and aberration, we are referring to the physiological refractivity of the conduction system; it is impossible for the heart to conduct normally when it has not recovered from another impulse. This is considered normal and prevents the heart from contracting too rapidly; however, when an impulse should be able to be conducted and is not, it is considered AV block.

In second degree AV block Wenckebach or Mobitz I, the conduction of sinus or supraventricular impulses to the ventricles becomes increasingly more difficult, causing progressively longer PR intervals until a P wave is not conducted. The pause following the dropped P wave enables the AV node to recover, and the following P wave is conducted with a normal or slightly shorter PR interval. The R-R interval in each sequence becomes progressively shorter until the pause occurs. A junctional or ventricular escape beat may terminate the pause.

The following criteria are used for recognition of second degree AV block Wenckebach:

1. PR progressively lengthens until a P wave is not conducted.
2. The R-R cycle shortens before the pause.
3. The P-P intervals are constant.

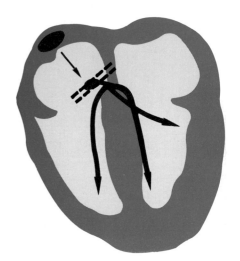

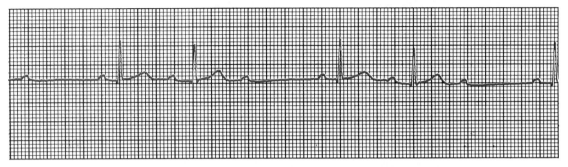

Sinus Rhythm With Second Degree AV Block Wenckebach

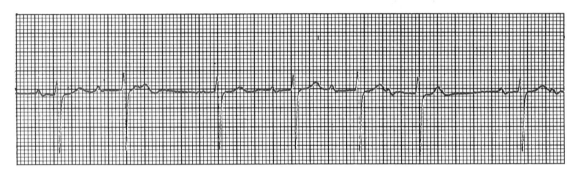

Sinus Rhythm With Second Degree AV Block Wenckebach

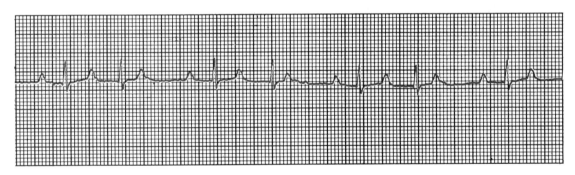

Sinus Rhythm With Second Degree AV Block Wenckebach

SECOND DEGREE AV BLOCK MOBITZ AND HIGH GRADE AV BLOCK

In second degree AV block Mobitz, the conduction of sinus or supraventricular impulses to the ventricles occurs with intermittent block of some of the P waves. The PR interval is of constant duration, and no more than one P wave in a row is blocked. The ventricular rate is slower than the atrial rate because of the blocked P waves, and the ventricular pauses are often terminated by junctional or ventricular escape beats.

The following criteria are used for recognition of second degree AV block Mobitz:

1. The PR interval is of constant duration.
2. There is one blocked sinus P wave for each QRS.

High grade AV block is the conduction of sinus or supraventricular impulses to the ventricles with intermittent block of more than one sinus P wave in a row. The ventricular rate is slower than the atrial rate because of the blocked P waves. Atrial fibrillation and flutter with high grade AV block produce long ventricular pauses that are often terminated by junctional or ventricular escape beats or rhythms.

The following criteria are used for recognition of high grade AV block:

1. The PR interval is of constant duration.
2. There are two or more blocked sinus P waves for each QRS.
3. In atrial fibrillation or flutter, long ventricular pauses are present.

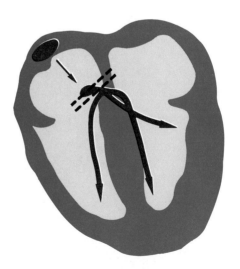

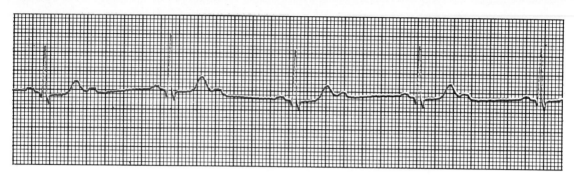

Sinus Rhythm With Second Degree AV Block Mobitz

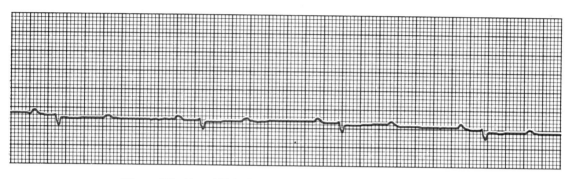

Sinus Rhythm With Second Degree AV Block Mobitz

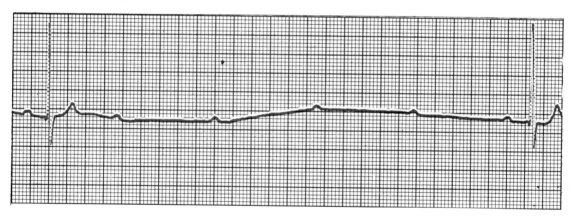

Sinus Bradycardia With High Grade AV Block

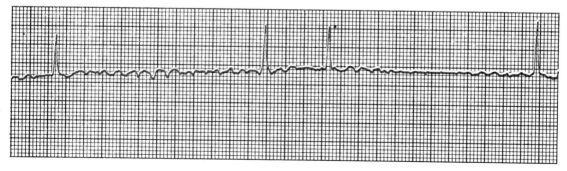

Atrial Fibrillation With High Grade AV Block

COMPLETE AV BLOCK

In complete or third degree AV block the atria and ventricles beat independently, each under the control of a separate pacemaking focus. The PR interval is constantly changing because the P waves and QRS complexes bear no relationship to one another and conduction between the atria and ventricles does not occur. The atria are under the control of a sinus or supraventricular pacemaker, and the ventricles are rescued by either a junctional or ventricular escape rhythm.

The following criteria are used for recognition of complete AV block:

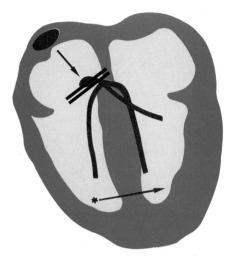

1. The PR interval varies because the P wave bears no relationship to the QRS.
2. There is no conduction between the atria and the ventricles.
3. The atria are under the control of a sinus or supraventricular focus, and the ventricles are controlled by either a junctional or ventricular escape rhythm.
4. In atrial fibrillation the ventricular rate is slow and regular due to a junctional or ventricular escape rhythm.

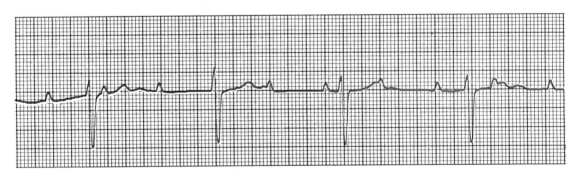

Sinus Rhythm With Complete Heart Block and Accelerated Idioventricular Rhythm

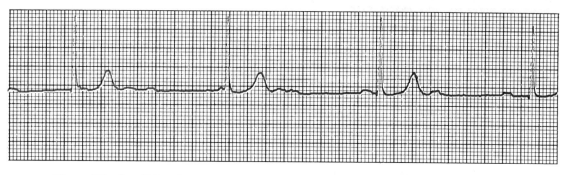

Sinus Rhythm With Complete Heart Block and Junctional Escape Rhythm

SINOATRIAL BLOCK

Sinoatrial (SA) block is a conduction disturbance between the sinus node and the surrounding atrial tissue that can cause delay or block in the conduction of sinus impulses to the atria.

Second degree SA block Wenckebach is characterized by a ventricular pause that is preceded by progressively shorter P-P intervals, and which measures less than twice the length of the preceding P-P interval.

The following criteria are used for recognition of second degree SA block Wenckebach:

1. P-P cycles are progressively shorter before a ventricular pause.
2. The ventricular pause measures less than twice the length of the preceding P-P cycle.
3. P-QRS-T is absent during the ventricular pause.

Second degree SA block Mobitz is characterized by a P-P cycle of constant duration and a ventricular pause that measure two, three, or more times the length of the normal P-P interval. Junctional or ventricular escape beats may interrupt the ventricular pauses.

The following criteria are used for recognition of second degree SA block Mobitz:

1. The P-P interval is of constant duration.
2. The ventricular pause measure two, three, or more times the length of the normal P-P interval.
3. P-QRS-T is missing during the ventricular pause.

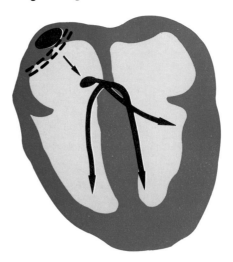

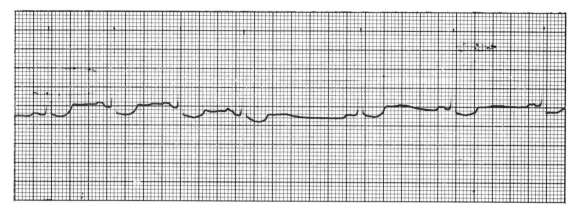

Sinus Rhythm With Second Degree SA Block Wenckebach

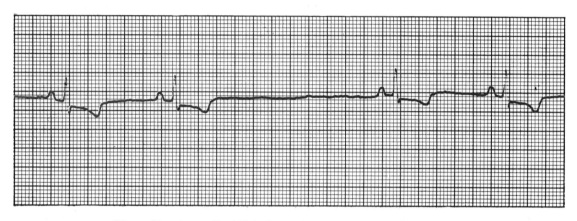

Sinus Bradycardia With Second Degree SA Block Mobitz

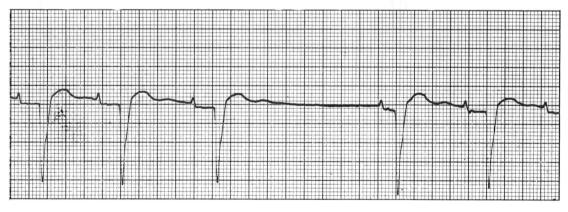

Sinus Rhythm With First Degree AV Block and Second Degree SA Block Mobitz (The pause is terminated by a junctional escape beat.)

WOLFF–PARKINSON–WHITE SYNDROME

In the Wolff–Parkinson–White syndrome (WPW), an accessory conduction pathway is present between the atria and the ventricles. WPW is characterized by a shortened PR interval as the impulse conducts rapidly to the ventricles via an accessory pathway, a slurring of the initial portion of the QRS (delta wave), and often a widened QRS complex. There will be varying degrees of slurring and widening, depending on each conduction pathway's contribution to ventricular activation.

DELTA WAVES

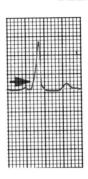

**Positive
Delta Wave**

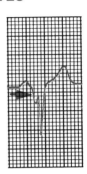

**Negative
Delta Wave**

WPW is associated with supraventricular tachycardias that tend to mimic ventricular tachycardia because the QRS is so wide.

The following criteria are used for recognition of WPW syndrome:

1. The PR interval is short.
2. A delta wave exists.
3. There is a variation in the widening of the QRS complex.
4. There are intermittent episodes of supraventricular tachycardia.

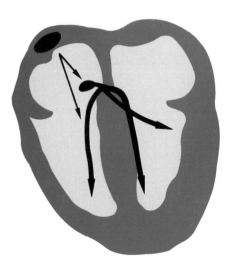

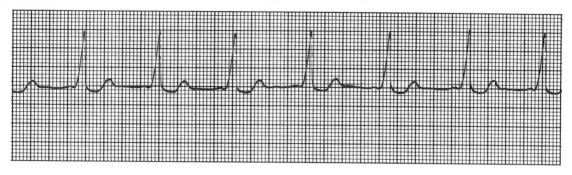

Sinus Rhythm With WPW

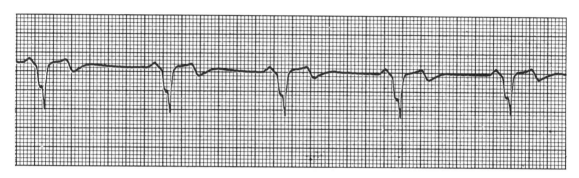

Sinus Bradycardia With WPW

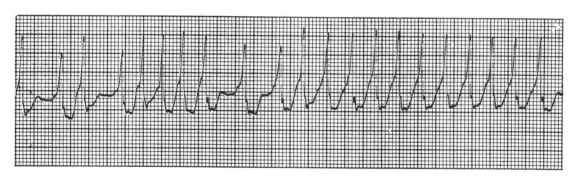

Atrial Fibrillation and WPW Mimicking Ventricular Tachycardia

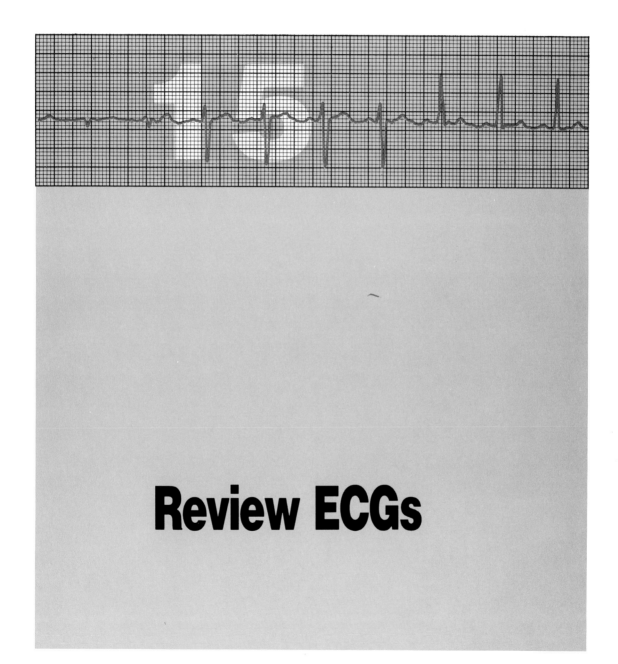

Review ECGs

On the following pages is a collection of 25 ECGs illustrating the ECG abnormalities discussed in the preceding chapters. The review ECGs will enable you to practice your interpretation skills and to determine correct differential diagnoses. The answers will be found at the end of the chapter.

REVIEW ECG 1

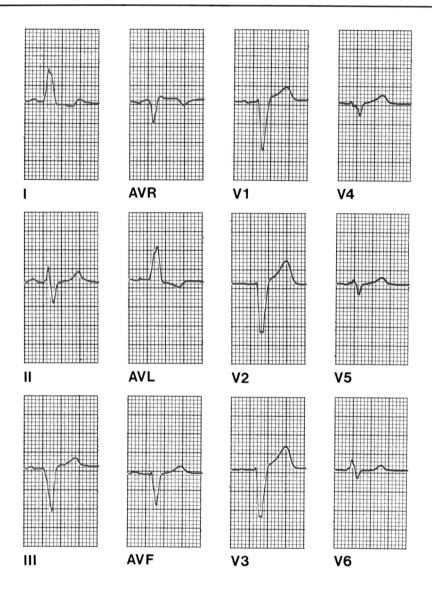

I AVR V1 V4

II AVL V2 V5

III AVF V3 V6

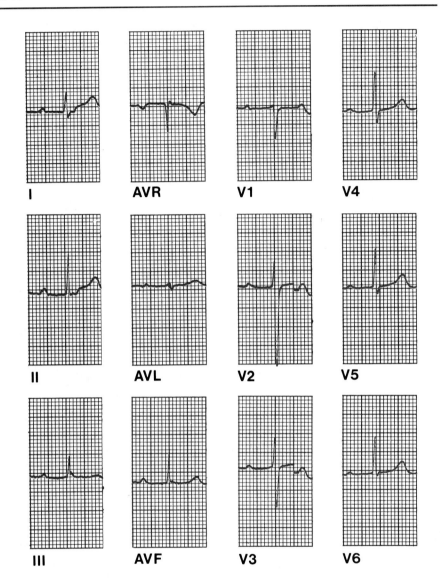

I AVR V1 V4

II AVL V2 V5

III AVF V3 V6

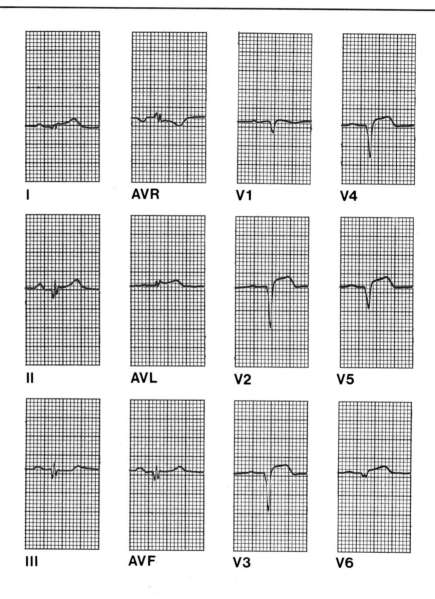

I AVR V1 V4

II AVL V2 V5

III AVF V3 V6

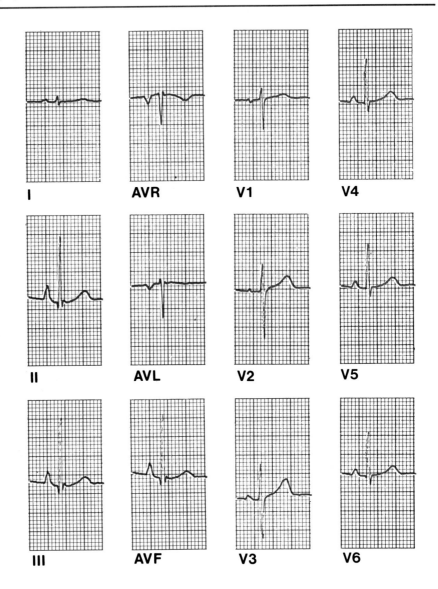

I   AVR   V1   V4

II   AVL   V2   V5

III   AVF   V3   V6

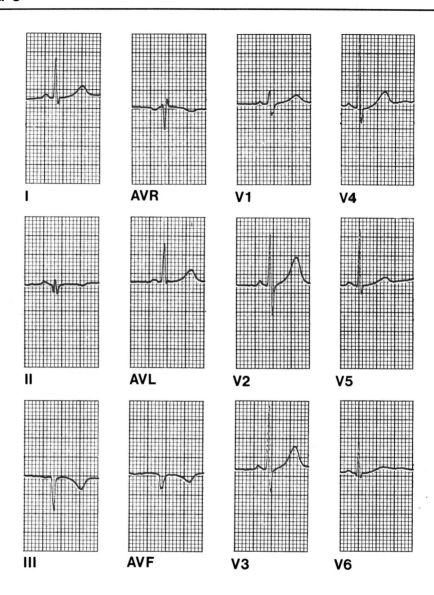

I AVR V1 V4

II AVL V2 V5

III AVF V3 V6

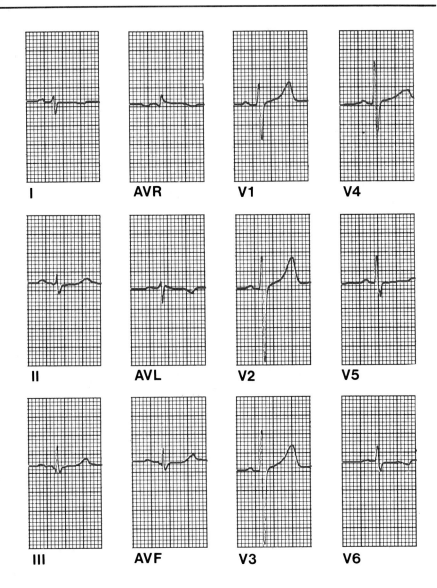

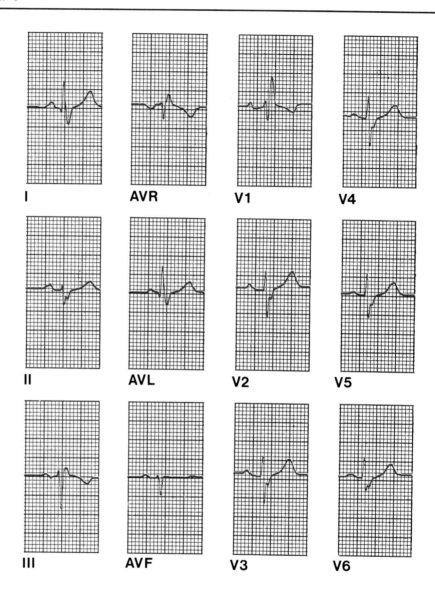

I   AVR   V1   V4

II   AVL   V2   V5

III   AVF   V3   V6

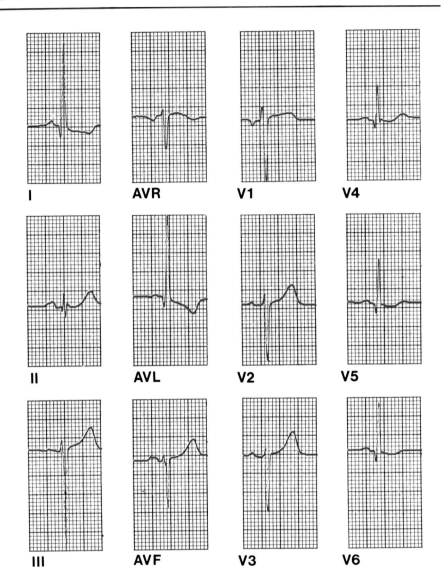

I AVR V1 V4

II AVL V2 V5

III AVF V3 V6

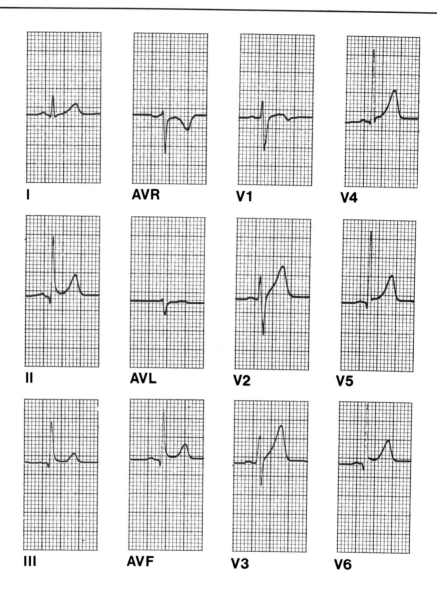

I AVR V1 V4

II AVL V2 V5

III AVF V3 V6

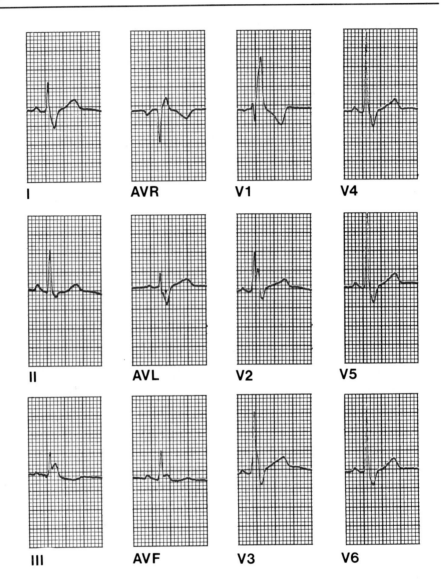

I AVR V1 V4

II AVL V2 V5

III AVF V3 V6

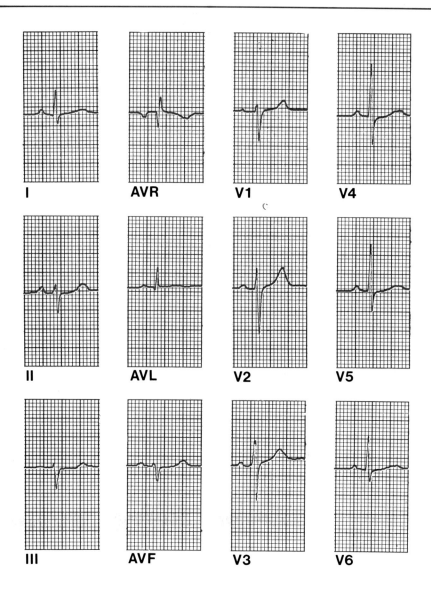

I AVR V1 V4

II AVL V2 V5

III AVF V3 V6

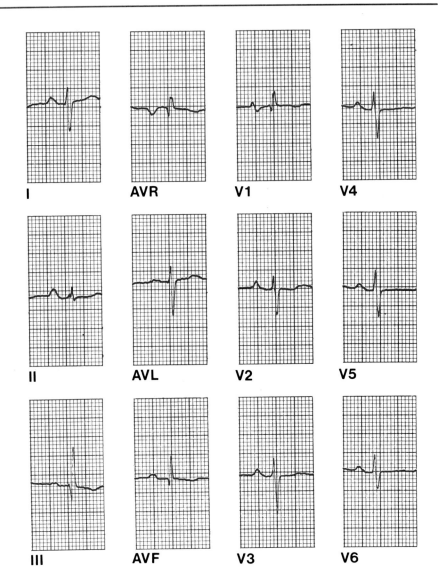

I   AVR   V1   V4

II   AVL   V2   V5

III   AVF   V3   V6

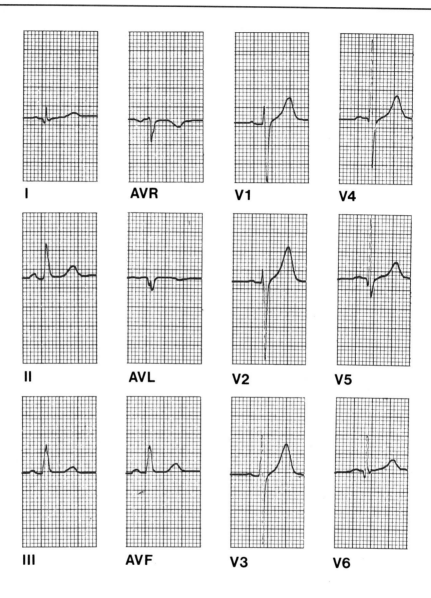

I   AVR   V1   V4

II   AVL   V2   V5

III   AVF   V3   V6

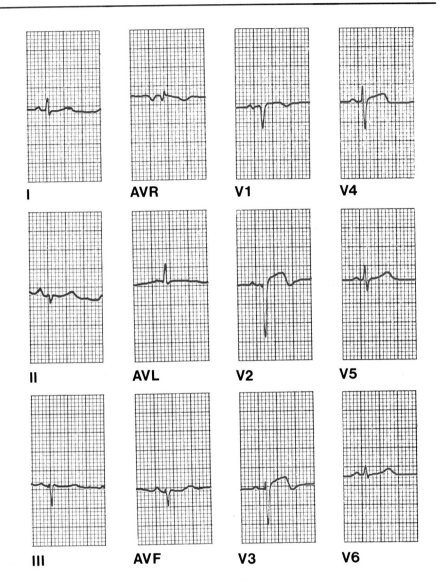

I AVR V1 V4

II AVL V2 V5

III AVF V3 V6

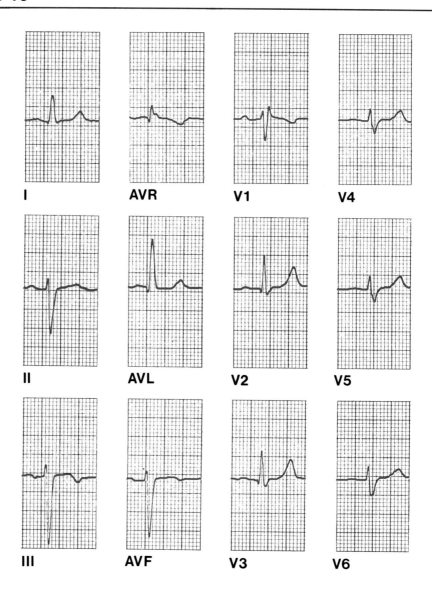

I AVR V1 V4

II AVL V2 V5

III AVF V3 V6

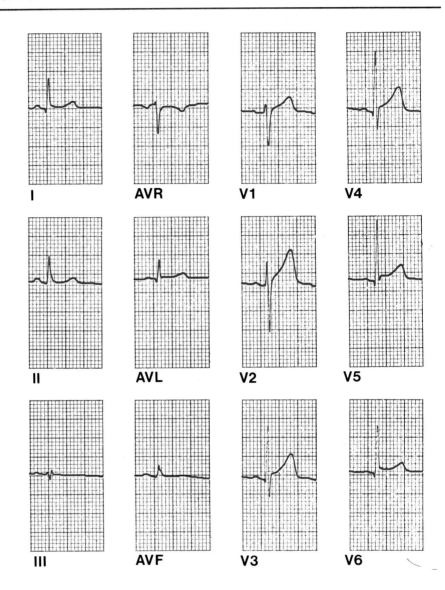

I AVR V1 V4

II AVL V2 V5

III AVF V3 V6

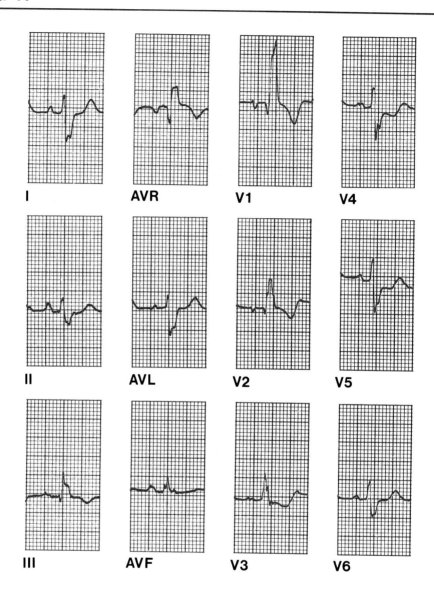

I   AVR   V1   V4

II   AVL   V2   V5

III   AVF   V3   V6

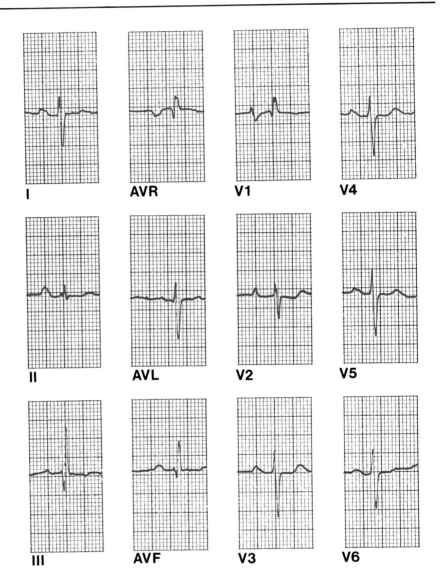

I   AVR   V1   V4

II   AVL   V2   V5

III   AVF   V3   V6

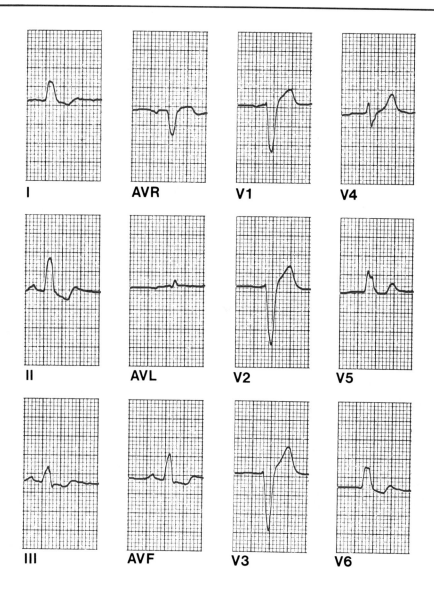

I AVR V1 V4

II AVL V2 V5

III AVF V3 V6

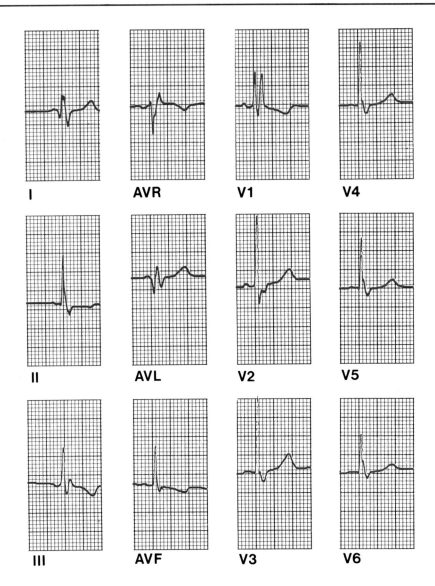

I   AVR   V1   V4

II   AVL   V2   V5

III   AVF   V3   V6

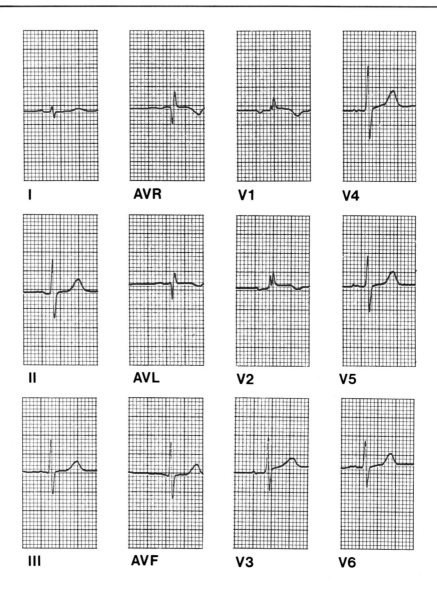

I   AVR   V1   V4

II   AVL   V2   V5

III   AVF   V3   V6

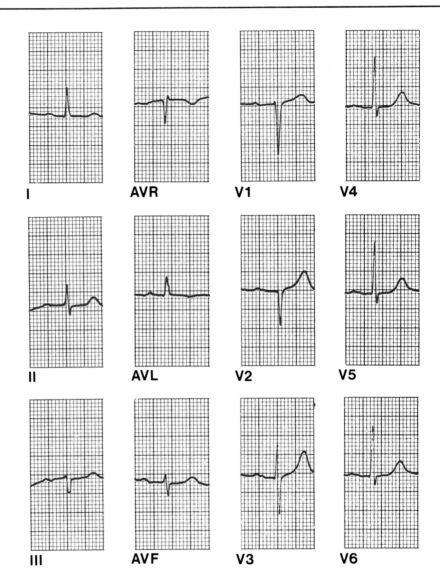

I AVR V1 V4

II AVL V2 V5

III AVF V3 V6

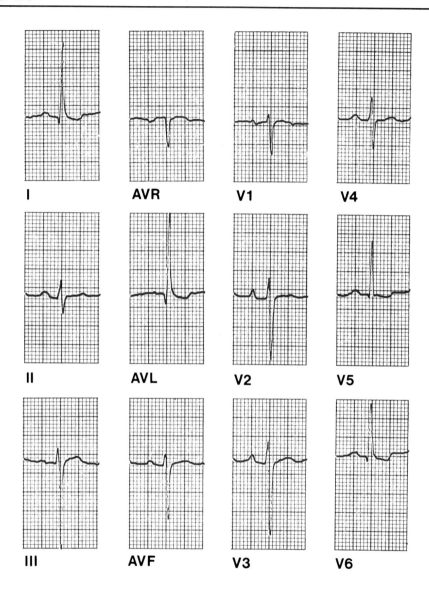

I   AVR   V1   V4

II   AVL   V2   V5

III   AVF   V3   V6

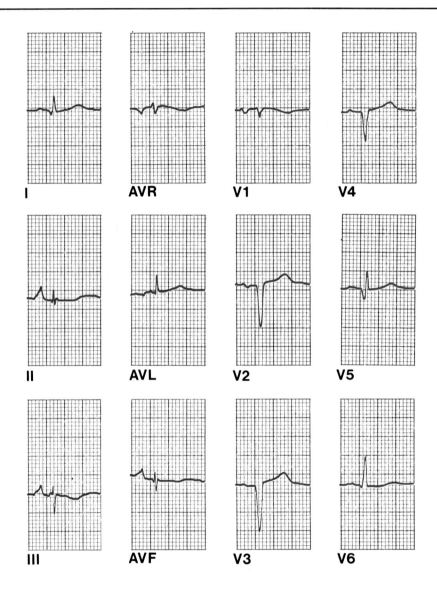

I AVR V1 V4

II AVL V2 V5

III AVF V3 V6

REVIEW ECG 25

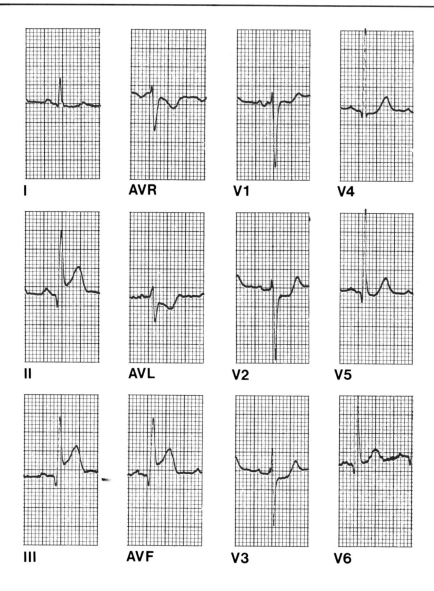

I AVR V1 V4

II AVL V2 V5

III AVF V3 V6

REVIEW ECG ANSWERS

1. Left bundle branch block
2. First degree AV block
3. Acute anterior, lateral, and old inferior myocardial infarction (MI)
4. Right atrial hypertrophy
5. Inferior and posterior MI, age indeterminate
6. Left posterior hemiblock
7. Left anterior hemiblock and right bundle branch block
8. Left atrial hypertrophy and left ventricular hypertrophy
9. Early repolarization vs. pericarditis
10. Right bundle branch block
11. Left anterior hemiblock
12. First degree AV block, left atrial hypertrophy, and right ventricular hypertrophy
13. Old lateral MI
14. Left anterior hemiblock and anterior septal MI, age indeterminate
15. First degree AV block, left anterior hemiblock, and right bundle branch block
16. Early repolarization vs. pericarditis
17. Left posterior hemiblock and right bundle branch block
18. First degree AV block, left atrial hypertrophy, and right ventricular hypertrophy
19. Left bundle branch block
20. Accelerated AV conduction, right bundle branch block, and old lateral MI
21. Right ventricular hypertrophy
22. First degree AV block and old anterior septal MI
23. Left ventricular hypertrophy
24. Biatrial hypertrophy and old anterior and lateral MI
25. Left ventricular hypertrophy and acute inferior MI with reciprocal ST depression

BIBLIOGRAPHY

Chung E: Electrocardiography, 2nd ed. Philadelphia, Harper & Row, 1980

Dubin D: Rapid Interpretation of EKG's, 3rd ed. Tampa, Cover Publishing, 1978

Goldman MJ: Principles of Clinical Electrocardiography, 11th ed. Los Altos, Lange, 1982

Mangiola S, Ritota M: Cardiac Arrhythmias. Philadelphia, JB Lippincott, 1974

Marriott H: Practical Electrocardiography, 7th ed. Baltimore, Williams & Wilkins, 1983

Netter F: Ciba Collection of Medical Illustrations, Vol 5, The Heart. Rochester, Case–Hoyt, 1981

Rosenbaum M, Elizari M, Lazzari J: The Hemiblocks. Oldsmar, Florida, Tampa Tracings, 1970

INDEX

Index

Index

348